Neurology for Nurses

NEUROLOGY FOR NURSES

J Bickerton, B.A. S.R.N. S.C.M. R.N.T.

Senior Tutor, Portsmouth District School of Nursing
Examiner to the General Nursing Council of England & Wales.

J Small, S.R.N. R.M.N. R.N.T.

Senior Tutor, Portsmouth District School of Nursing
Examiner to the General Nursing Council of England & Wales.

WILLIAM HEINEMANN MEDICAL BOOKS LTD

LONDON

First published 1981
© J. Bickerton and J. Small 1981

ISBN 0 433 02830 0

Printed and bound in Great Britain by
REDWOOD BURN LIMITED
Trowbridge & Esher

CONTENTS

Chapter		Page
1	The planes of the body	1
2	The neurone	3
3	Introduction to the central nervous system	9
4	The forebrain	11
5	The thalamus	17
6	The basal nuclei	19
7	The hypothalamus	21
8	The neurohypophysis (posterior pituitary)	27
9	The brain stem	29
10	The cerebellum	33
11	The meninges	35
12	The ventricles	37
13	Cerebrospinal fluid	39
14	Arterial supply of the brain	41
15	Venous drainage of the brain	43
16	The spinal cord	45
17	Ascending sensory tracts	47
18	Descending motor tracts	49
19	The reflex arc	51
20	An introduction to the peripheral nervous system	53
21	The spinal nerves	55
22	The cranial nerves	57
23	The nerves of the upper limb	59
24	The nerves of the lower limb	61
25	Sight	63
26	Hearing	65
27	Balance	67
28	Smell and taste	69
29	Touch	71
30	The autonomic nervous system	73
31	Neurological examination	77
32	Neurological investigations	83
33	Neurological observations	89
34	Care of the unconscious patient	91
35	Care of the paralysed patient	95
36	Multiple sclerosis	101
37	Cerebro vascular accident	113
38	Brain tumours	123
39	Head injury	131
40	Epilepsy	143
31	Parkinsonism	153
42	Meningitis	161
43	Encephalitis	167
44	Subarachnoid haemorrhage	169
45	Lesions of the spinal cord	177

46 Acute poliomyelitis   179
47 Spina bifida   187
48 Hydrocephalus   191
49 Peripheral neuritis   193
50 The trigeminal and facial nerves   201
51 Menières disease   203
52 Headache and migraine   205

PREFACE

Many nurses, both in training and when qualified, have difficulty in understanding the nervous system. This book is an attempt to make the subject as clear as possible, using the nursing model.

It is aimed primarily at the student nurse in training who seeks further knowledge, but may also be seen as an introduction to the subject for those taking a post-basic nursing course in neurology.

We would like to thank all those who have been involved in the making of this book, particularly our students, who have been the stimulus, and our publishers, who have guided us through its preparation.

J.B.
J.S.

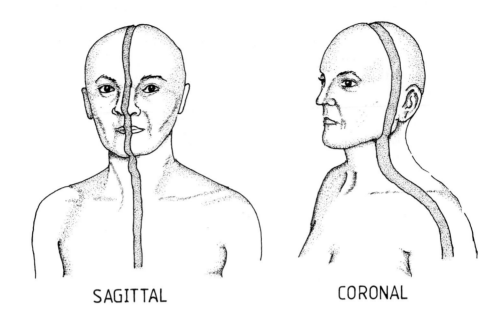

SAGITTAL   CORONAL

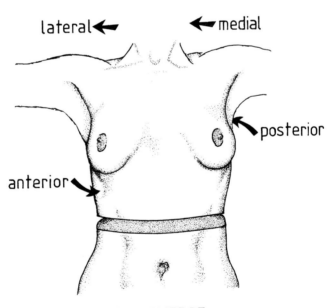

lateral ←   ← medial

posterior

anterior

TRANSVERSE

1 The planes of the body

When considering the nervous system anatomically it is necessary to divide the body diagrammatically along different planes in order to look at the various parts from different directions. The following are the different orientations and planes used in this book.

Anterior (ventral) surface	–	towards or at the front
Posterior (dorsal) surface	–	towards or at the back
Lateral	–	away from the midline, on the side.
Medial	–	towards the midline.
Sagittal (median) section	–	dividing the body from top to bottom into a right and left part.
Coronal (frontal) section	–	dividing the front from the back, i.e. vertically at right angles to the sagittal section.
Transverse	–	dividing the upper part of the body from the lower. A horizontal section through the body.

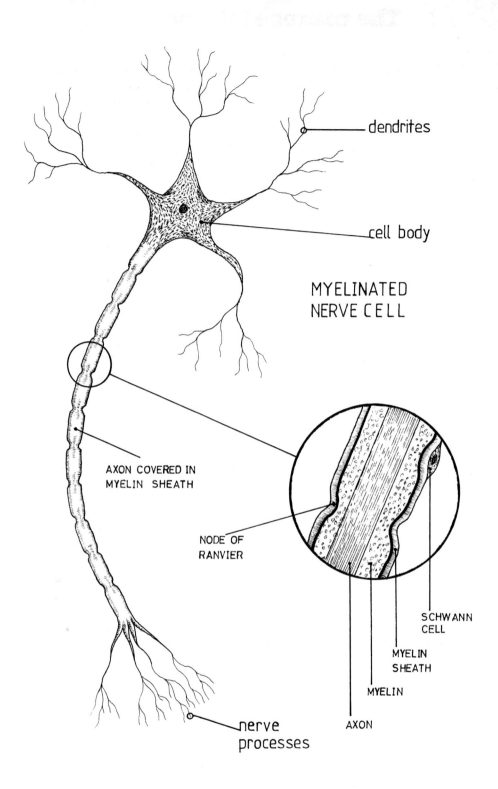

dendrites

cell body

MYELINATED
NERVE CELL

AXON COVERED IN
MYELIN SHEATH

NODE OF
RANVIER

SCHWANN
CELL

MYELIN
SHEATH

MYELIN

AXON

nerve
processes

2 The neurone

The neurone or nerve cell is the functional unit of the nervous system. It consists of a **cell body** and a number of **nerve fibres.** The function of the neurone is to carry information in the form of nerve impulses from one point to another.

As with any other cell in the body, cytoplasm forms the major part, with a nucleus at its centre. Surrounding the nucleus are the Nissl granules which contain RNA and are thought to produce protein for the cells. The cells come in a variety of shapes, and compared with other cells in the body are relatively large. For example the red blood cell is about 7·5 microns in diameter whereas the neurone may vary from 10–100 microns. The nerve cell body is essential for the life of the nerve and if it is destroyed it cannot regenerate.

Attached to the cell body are the nerve fibres. These are of two types: the **dendrites,** which are short, branching fibres receiving information, of which there may be one or more, and the **axon** which may be short or more than a metre long and of varying thickness. The axon transmits information away from the nerve cell. It may give off branches along its length, and at its far end has several small branches. Within these nerve endings are vesicles containing chemical transmitter substances, necessary to produce another impulse in the connecting neurone, or to act on the muscle cell.

Those axons found in the peripheral nervous system and in reflex arcs, those connecting the spinal cord and cerebellum, and the motor fibres to the muscles, are all surrounded by a fatty sheath, the **myelin sheath,** and are therefore called myelinated nerves. This sheath is wound around the axon in a spiral fashion and is much thicker than the axon itself. It acts as an insulator preventing impulses jumping across to the neighbouring nerves. The myelin sheath is interrupted at intervals along its length, allowing the outer membrane, the neurilemma, to dip down and touch the axon. These dips are called the **nodes of Ranvier.** The neurilemma and Schwann cell are present in non-myelinated neurones as well. They are both necessary for the regeneration of the nerve fibre. Surrounding the whole is connective tissue, which binds the neurones together to form a nerve. Non-myelinated nerves are found in the autonomic nervous system.

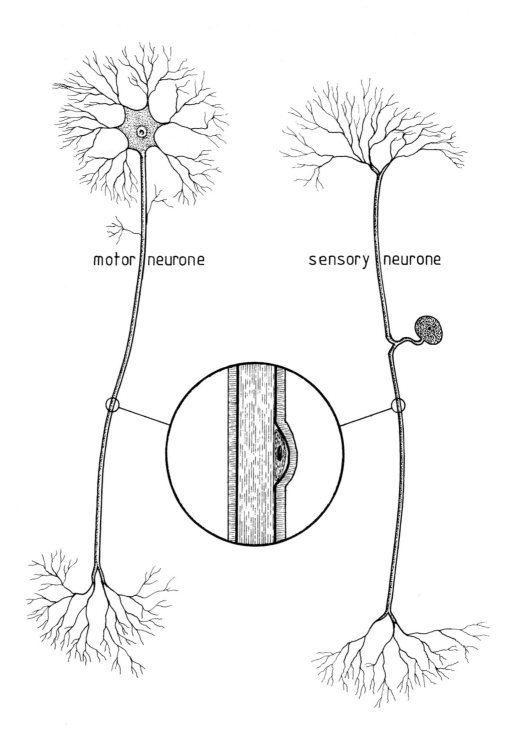

motor neurone   sensory neurone

The **motor neurone** has its cell body at one end of the axon. It transmits information from the brain and spinal cord to the muscles and glands. **Sensory neurones** have the cell body to one side, with dendrites and axon coming off a short process. They receive information from receptors and send it to the spinal cord and brain. Association neurones link one neurone to another. In the nervous system there are also cells which do not receive or transmit information; they are the connective tissue of the nervous system and support, feed and repair the neurones. In the brain and spinal cord they are called **neuroglia,** and in the peripheral nervous system, the **Schwann cells.**

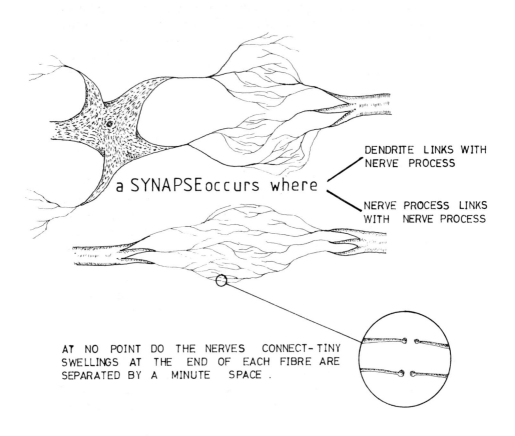

a SYNAPSE occurs where

DENDRITE LINKS WITH NERVE PROCESS

NERVE PROCESS LINKS WITH NERVE PROCESS

AT NO POINT DO THE NERVES CONNECT- TINY SWELLINGS AT THE END OF EACH FIBRE ARE SEPARATED BY A MINUTE SPACE .

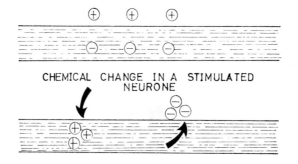

CHEMICAL CHANGE IN A STIMULATED NEURONE

The synapse

The nerve endings of the axon, with their vesicles, will connect with the dendrites or cell body of another neurone, or with a muscle cell or gland. The junction of one neurone with another it is called a synapse. Several neurones may be involved in the synapse and any one neurone is likely to link up with many others. Under the electron microscope it can be seen that there is a minute gap between the synaptic knobs of the axon and the dendrites or cell body with which they are linking.

The nerve impulse

As has already been said the function of a neurone is to carry nerve impulses. These have been likened to a 'wave of negativity' along the axon of a neurone. Information is picked up by receptor cells. This may be in a chemical form as in the eyes (*see* p. 63), or a physical form from pressure on the skin or sound waves on the ear drums, or it may start off as an electrical stimulus from another nerve. Sometimes the receptor is part of the neurone, sometimes it links with it. In either case the information is transformed into an electrical impulse, whatever causes the original stimulation.

When a neurone is at rest the cytoplasm in the axon is rich in potassium, but because it also has a large number of protein molecules and some chloride the membrane is negative on the inside. The tissue fluid bathing the outside of the membrane is rich in sodium, with some chloride. It is therefore positive. When the neurone is stimulated to a sufficient degree the membrane becomes permeable to sodium which enters the axon. This alters the balance between positive and negative ions across the surface membrane of the axon. The result is that this section of the axon has negative ions on the outside of its surface membrane and positive ions inside. This change happens section by section along the whole length of the neurone. Until the membrane has been restored to its normal state, another impulse is unable to pass along it.

This process is speeded up in the myelinated nerves because the impulse is able to jump from one node of Ranvier to the next. It is also quicker in the thicker nerves. When the impulse reaches the nerve endings the chemical transmitter substance is released which then initiates another impulse in the next neurone, or stimulates a muscle to contract or a gland to secrete. An impulse will not be triggered off in a neurone unless the stimulus is of sufficient strength.

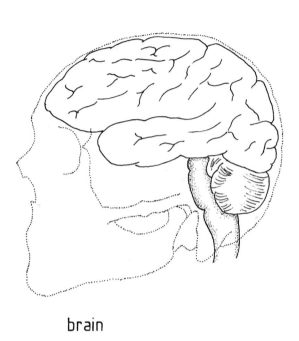

brain

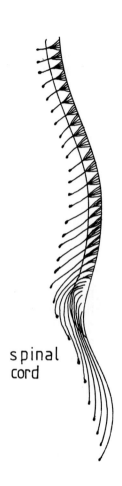

spinal
cord

3 Introduction to the central nervous system

The central nervous system consists of the **brain,** which is within the cranial cavity, and the **spinal cord** contained within the vertebral column.

The brain

This includes the two cerebral hemispheres, the cerebellum, the thalamus, the basal ganglia, the hypothalamus, the midbrain, pons, and medulla oblongata. All of these have a large number of nerve cells and their fibres. The internal capsule and the corpus callosum are specific groups of nerve fibres within the brain. Also within the substance of the brain are the ventricles and the tissues secreting and absorbing cerebrospinal fluid.

The spinal cord

This is continuous with the brain. It has nerve cells at the centre and fibres surrounding these. The latter include sensory fibres bringing information from the peripheral nervous system to the brain, and motor fibres taking information from the brain to the peripheral nervous system.

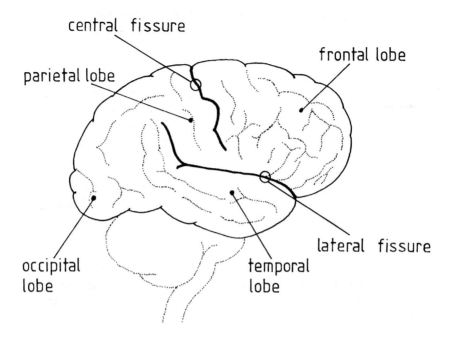

central fissure

frontal lobe

parietal lobe

occipital
lobe

temporal
lobe

lateral fissure

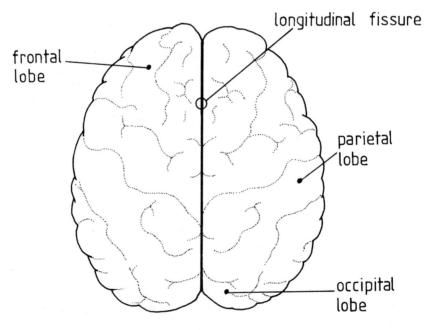

longitudinal fissure

frontal
lobe

parietal
lobe

occipital
lobe

4 The forebrain

The forebrain consists of the two **cerebral hemispheres**, which almost fill the skull, the **thalamus** and the **hypothalamus**, with associated nerve fibres.

The cerebral hemispheres
These are separated from one another by the median **longitudinal fissure** into which the dura mater (*see* p. 35) dips. Although almost entirely separated from each other by this fissure, they are linked at the base of it by nerve fibres called the **corpus callosum.** This ensures that information reaching one side of the brain is transmitted to the other, and they can therefore work together and not separately. Such bundles of fibres are called commissures.

Although the two hemispheres appear almost identical, one of them is dominant. In right-handed people this is normally the left hemisphere. It is on the dominant side that the centre for speech, and the thought processes required for it, are found. Each hemisphere receives information from, and controls, the opposite side of the body. This means that damage to the left hemisphere in a right-handed person will result in disturbance of speech and right-sided paralysis.

The cerebral hemispheres also have two other fissures which are not so marked as the longitudinal fissure. The deeper **lateral fissure** separates the frontal region from the temporal. The **central fissure** lies between the frontal and parietal lobes. Apart from these deeper fissures the cerebral hemispheres have many convolutions, so increasing the surface area and accomodating many more neurones. These convolutions are arranged in the same manner in all normal human brains. The convolutions are called gyri (sing. gyrus) and the dips or fissures are called sulci (sing. sulcus).

The cerebral cortex
The outer surface of the cerebral hemispheres is called the cerebral cortex and consists mainly of nerve cell bodies, although there are some supporting cells (neuroglia) and a few nerve fibres. Because it is predominantly nerve cells it has a slightly darker look to it and is called **grey matter.** Although there are nerve cell bodies throughout the central nervous system the majority are in the cerebral cortex. Because the nerve cells are on the convoluted outer surface of the brain there are a greater number. Although there are groups of nerve cells within the substance of the brain this area is mainly composed of nerve fibres, or white matter. The cerebral cortex is not essential for survival, but it is necessary to live life in a meaningful way. We see what can happen if the cerebral cortex is not functioning normally in patients who are brain damaged.

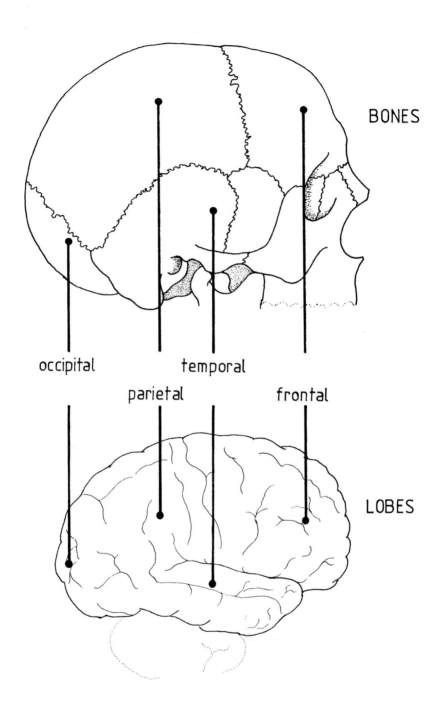

BONES

occipital

parietal

temporal

frontal

LOBES

In order to aid description, the cerebral cortex is divided into lobes which take their names from the skull bones overlying them. The area in front of the central fissure is called the **frontal lobe,** and the area immediately behind it is the **parietal lobe.** The posterior area is called the **occipital lobe.** The area below the lateral fissure is called the **temporal lobe.** There is no anatomical division between these lobes, association fibres linking one area with another in the same hemisphere.

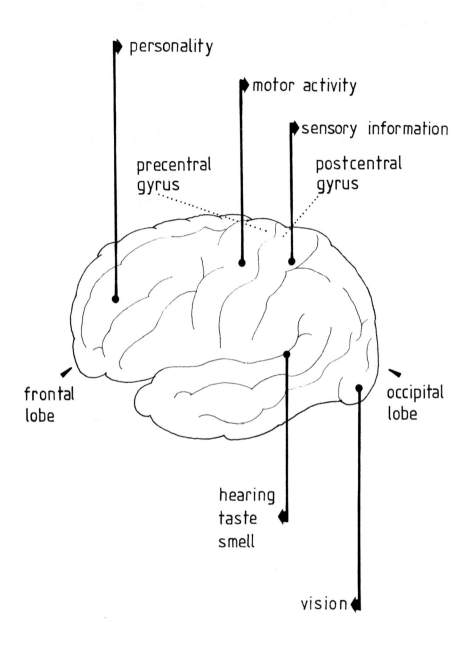

personality

motor activity

sensory information

precentral
gyrus

postcentral
gyrus

frontal
lobe

occipital
lobe

hearing
taste
smell

vision

It has been possible by means of experiments with animals and electrical stimulation of exposed human brain to map out various functions in the cortex. However there are large areas which do not appear to have specific functions. These areas do have a major part to play in the higher activities of the brain such as the storage of information, intelligence and imagination.

The frontal lobe plays a major part in personality, and appears to exert some control over our more primitive instincts. Its most posterior part contains a strip immediately in front of the central fissure which is called the **precentral gyrus** and is responsible for initiating motor activity. The various parts of the body involved in motor activity are represented in this area. Those parts such as the thumb which have very precise movement are represented by a much larger area in the brain than, for example, the trunk. The relationship between areas represented in this narrow strip in the brain corresponds with that between the actual members of the body, except that the representation is upside down. Adjacent to the precentral gyrus is the premotor area. This area modifies motor activity.

In the parietal lobe there is a similar strip immediately behind the central fissure which is called the **postcentral gyrus.** This is the receptive area for sensory information. As with the motor area the various parts of the body experiencing the sensations of touch, temperature etc., are represented on this strip, the size of the representative area reflecting the sensitivity of the part, so that lips and finger tips have a relatively larger representation in the brain than the trunk. It is in this area of the brain that the sensory and motor pathways link.

The occipital lobe contains the area of reception for information received via the eyes, and is able to interpret it. The temporal lobe receives information from the ears, taste receptors, and smell. On the dominant side where the frontal, parietal and temporal lobes meet is the area for speech.

To summarise the functions of the cortex:
1. Reception and interpretation of sensory stimuli
2. Reception and interpretation of vision
3. Reception and interpretation of hearing
4. Speech
5. Initiation of voluntary movement and motor activity
6. Storage of information therefore forming the basis of memory
7. Intelligence
8. Control of the lower parts of the nervous system

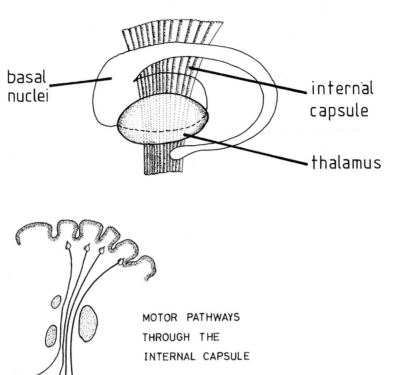

basal nuclei

internal capsule

thalamus

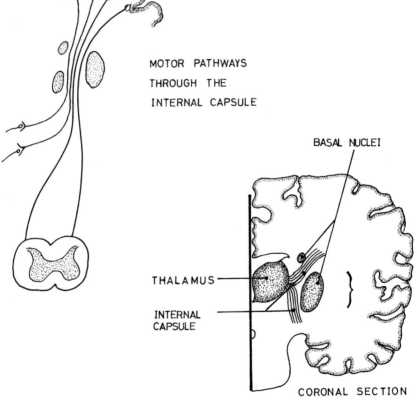

MOTOR PATHWAYS
THROUGH THE
INTERNAL CAPSULE

BASAL NUCLEI

THALAMUS

INTERNAL CAPSULE

CORONAL SECTION

the thalamus and adjacent structures

5 The thalamus

Within the substance of the cerebral hemispheres are groups of cells and their dendrites which form masses of grey matter, the thalamus and basal nuclei.

The thalamus
This consists of two oval masses of cells either side of the third ventricle. The lateral ventricles are just above. It is a relay centre through which all sensory information is passed and redirected, mainly to the cerebral cortex. It therefore receives information regarding pain, temperature and touch from receptors in the skin, position sense from receptors in muscles and tendons, and sensory impulses from some of the cranial nerves. It has links with the cerebellum and the basal nuclei, finally transmitting all the information to the cerebral cortex through the internal capsule.

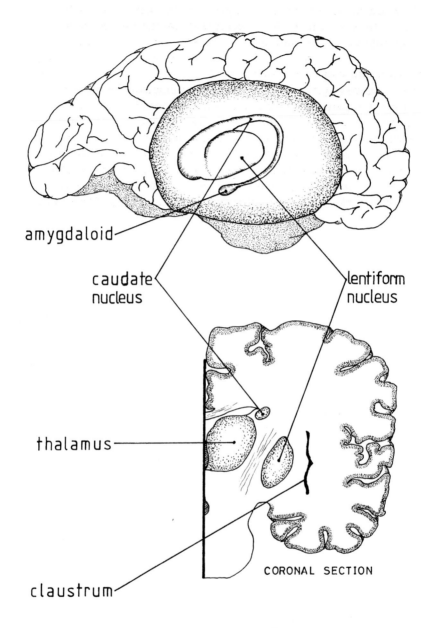

amygdaloid

caudate nucleus

lentiform nucleus

thalamus

claustrum

CORONAL SECTION

BASAL NUCLEI

6 The basal nuclei

The basal nuclei are masses of grey matter, not in the cortex but within the cerebral hemisphere, and separated from the thalami on each side by the internal capsule. They lie in close proximity to the lateral ventricles. They include the **corpus striatum**, the **amygdaloid body** and the **claustrum**. The corpus striatum consists of the caudate nucleus and the lentiform nucleus. The basal nuclei form the organising centre of the extra-pyramidal system. Information from the ears, thalamus, cerebellum and cerebral cortex is received here, so that body position, balance, muscle coordination all work together, modifying muscular contraction and movement as required. The basal nuclei are therefore important in maintaining posture, modifying reflex actions and ensuring that movements such as walking or other muscular skills are well co-ordinated and not erratic.

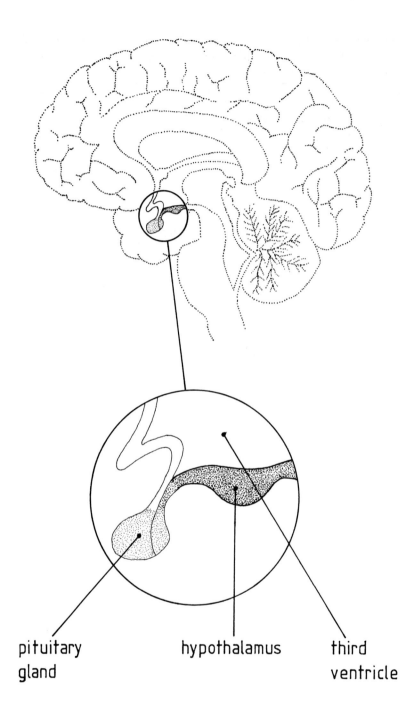

pituitary
gland

hypothalamus

third
ventricle

7 The hypothalamus

The hypothalamus is situated behind the optic chiasma and beneath the floor of the third ventricle. Its functions include the control of the posterior and anterior pituitary, the reticular formation, the autonomic nervous system, and body temperature.

Control of the posterior pituitary
Secretory nerve cells within the hypothalamus produce the hormones antidiuretic hormone (ADH) and oxtocin. These hormones travel via the nerve fibres to the posterior pituitary where they are stored (*see* p. 27).

Control of the anterior pituitary
The hypothalamus secretes a releasing factor for each of the hormones produced by the anterior pituitary, i.e. growth hormone, thyroid stimulating hormone, adrenocorticotrophic hormone (ACTH), and the gonadotrophic hormones (follicle stimulating hormone, luteinising hormone, and luteotrophic hormone). The releasing factor reaches the pituitary via portal vessels, and stimulates the production of the appropriate hormone.

the hypothalamus stimulates
the medulla

in response to emotion and change
of temperature

causing variations of

heart rate
respiration rate
blood pressure
temperature
metabolism

Action on the reticular formation

The hypothalamus, together with the cerebral cortex and basal ganglia, stimulates that part of the reticular formation (*see* p. 31) which accentuates movements originating in the cortex or in a reflex arc.

Control of the autonomic nervous system

In response to various emotions such as anger, fear, embarrassment, and grief, the hypothalamus sends nerve impulses to the medulla oblongata which contains the vital centres. In this way the heart rate, respiration, blood pressure temperature and metabolism can be adjusted to suit the situation.

Body temperature

The hypothalamus contains groups of nerve cells which are sensitive to changes in the temperature of the blood reaching them. It also receives information about body temperature via nerve impulses from temperature receptors in the skin. The core temperature of the body is that of the blood leaving the heart via the aorta. This is very similar to the temperature taken by mouth. Normal oral temperature is 36–37.5 °C. and varies slightly from one person to another. It is slightly higher in the evening than in the morning and in women it also varies during the menstrual cycle. This temperature is the result of a balance between the production of heat and its loss.

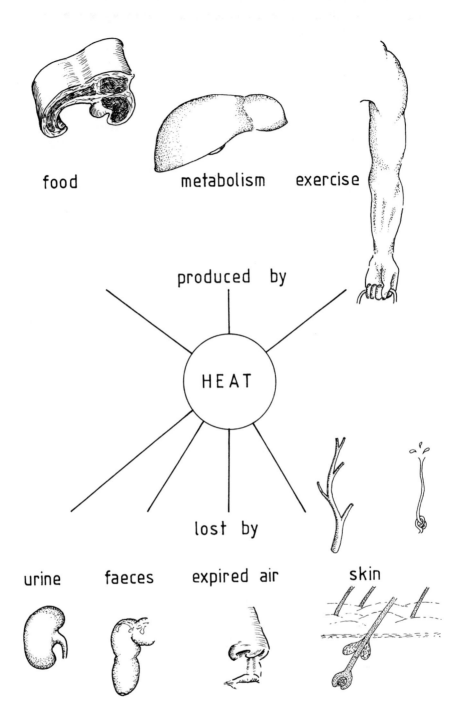

food   metabolism   exercise

produced by

HEAT

lost by

urine   faeces   expired air   skin

Heat is constantly being generated as a byproduct of various activities taking place within the body; principally these are the digestion of food, metabolic processes, particularly in the liver, and muscular activity, including shivering.

Atmospheric temperature, and the ingestion of hot food or drink also help to raise the core temperature. A rise in the temperature increases the rate of metabolic activity, so increasing body temperature even further and if there was no means of heat loss, death would soon occur.

Normal loss of heat from the body is through:

1. the skin, by (a) conduction of heat away from the body by cool currents of air; (b) radiation (loss of the heat to solid objects which come in contact with the body); and (c) evaporation, loss of heat in converting body sweat to water vapour.
2. expired air
3. urine
4. faeces.

We also take measures to control the body's temperature by the clothes we wear, increasing air currents with fans, and varying the amount of muscular activity.

A rise in the body temperature means that blood circulating in the region of the hypothalamus has a raised temperature, it will therefore stimulate the appropriate cells to act on the parasympathetic nervous system. Stimulation will also occur as a result of nerve impulses coming from the temperature receptors in the skin. Stimulation of the parasympathetic nervous system will cause:

1. vasodilatation of the blood vessels near the surface of the skin, so increasing the blood flow to that area, enabling heat to be lost by conduction and radiation;
2. increased production of sweat by the sweat glands so increasing evaporation.

A fall in the body temperature will act on other cells within the hypothalamus to stimulate the sympathetic nervous system, so causing:

1. vasoconstriction of blood vessels near the surface of the skin and therefore less heat loss;
2. shivering, producing heat.

This mechanism may be upset if there is damage to the hypothalamus as with some forms of head injury, or cerebral vascular accident. The control may be set at a higher level in a fever and certain drugs such as aspirin may also affect its activity.

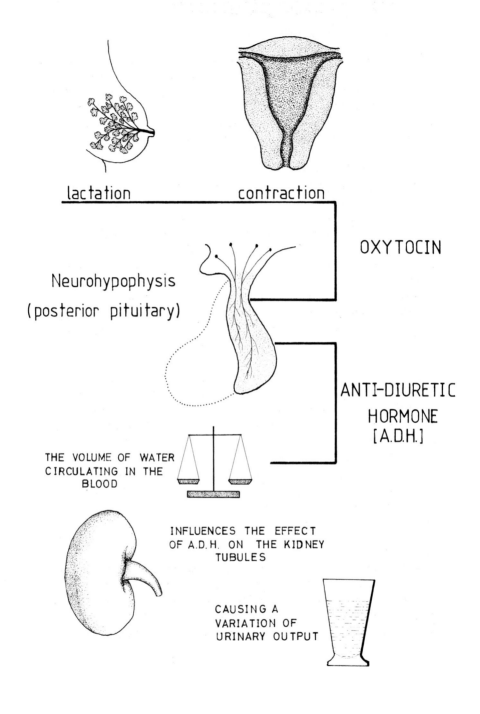

lactation   contraction

OXYTOCIN

Neurohypophysis
(posterior pituitary)

ANTI-DIURETIC
HORMONE
[A.D.H.]

THE VOLUME OF WATER
CIRCULATING IN THE
BLOOD

INFLUENCES THE EFFECT
OF A.D.H. ON THE KIDNEY
TUBULES

CAUSING A
VARIATION OF
URINARY OUTPUT

8 The neuro-hypophysis (posterior pituitary)

The pituitary gland, part of the endocrine system, also consists of nervous tissue. The posterior lobe although closely related anatomically to the anterior lobe, is functionally quite separate and is mainly nervous tissue. Nerve fibres connect the hypothalamus to the posterior lobe, so controlling its secretions. The two hormones secreted are **antidiuretic hormone (ADH)** and **oxytocin.**

Antidiuretic hormone

This hormone regulates the reabsorption of water by the kidney tubules. Large amounts of it also cause the blood pressure to rise, due to vasoconstriction of the blood vessels.

The hypothalamus controls the release of ADH according to the osmotic pressure of the blood circulating in that area. The hormone is secreted by the nerves passing between the hypothalamus and the pituitary. Both nerves and hormones are therefore involved. If the amount of fluid in the blood is decreased the osmotic pressure will increase. This increase of osmotic pressure will be picked up by receptors near the hypothalamus, which will in turn stimulate the secretory nerve fibres to produce more ADH. This acts on the distal convoluted tubule and collecting ducts of the nephron in the kidney, causing increased reabsorption of water and so lowering the osmotic pressure of the blood. The fall of the osmotic pressure will cause the hypothalamus to become less active once more, less ADH will be secreted and more urine will again be passed.

Many substances in common use inhibit the secretion of antidiuretic hormone and therefore act as diuretics, for example, coffee and alcohol. Destruction of the posterior pituitary results in diabetes inspididus, with excess urinary output, severe dehydration and electrolyte imbalance.

Oxytocin

This hormone is released in response to sensory stimuli from the vulva, uterus and breasts, which send nerve impulses to the hypothalamus, causing secretion of the hormone. It is important in child-birth, causing the uterus to contract during labour and after delivery it is responsible for the ejection of milk during lactation.

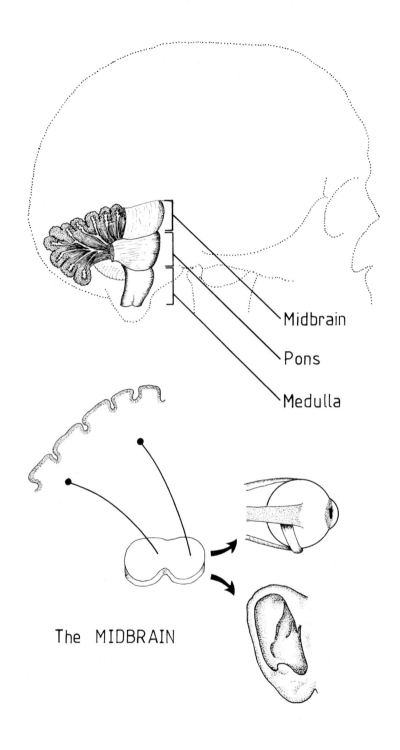

Midbrain

Pons

Medulla

The MIDBRAIN

9 The brain stem

The brain stem includes the **midbrain, pons** and **medulla oblongata.** All the cranial nerves except the olfactory and optic rise in this area. The ascending **reticular formation,** a network of cells and fibres, is also found here. The latter stretches from the medulla oblongata to the thalamus, and is responsible for keeping the cerebral cortex active. Damage to it will cause coma.

The midbrain
The smallest part of the brain stem consists mainly of motor and sensory nerve fibres connecting the cerebral hemispheres to the pons and cerebellum. It receives information from the ears and eyes and it is therefore involved in reflexes related to these organs. The nuclei of the third and fourth cranial nerves arise in the midbrain. It is therefore also involved in eye movement. The **red nucleus,** a relay point in the extrapyramidal system (p. 49), is in the midbrain and receives information from the basal ganglia and the hypothalamus, facilitating the action of the pyramidal system (p. 49).

The pons
The pons lies between the medulla and the midbrain and is joined to the cerebellum by the middle cerebellar peduncle. Between the pons and the cerebellum lies the fourth ventricle. The pons consists mainly of sensory and motor nerve fibres passing between the midbrain, cerebellum and medulla oblongata. The nerve cells of the fifth, sixth and seventh cranial nerves are scattered among the fibres. The fibres lying on top cross from one side to the other giving the appearance of a bridge, hence its name. Apart from transmitting sensory and motor information the pons also contains nuclei which form part of the respiratory centre with the medulla oblongata. The respiratory centre is sensitive to the level of carbon dioxide in the blood.

The medulla oblongata
The medulla oblongata consists of both cells and fibres, which are arranged similarly to those in the spinal cord, the cells or grey matter being on the inside and the fibres of white matter on the outside. It lies at the base of the skull just in front of the foramen magnum and links the pons and spinal cord. Collections of cells known as the **vital centres** are situated here. These include:
1. part of the respiratory centre which controls the rate and depth of respiration;
2. the vasomotor centre which controls the rate of the heart and the calibre of the blood vessels, and therefore blood pressure;
3. special centres for swallowing, vomiting, coughing, yawning, sneezing.

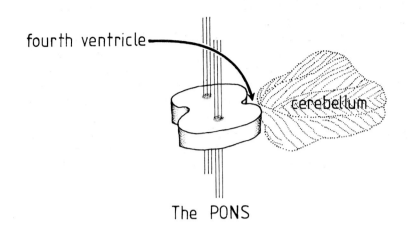

fourth ventricle

cerebellum

The PONS

The MEDULLA OBLONGATA

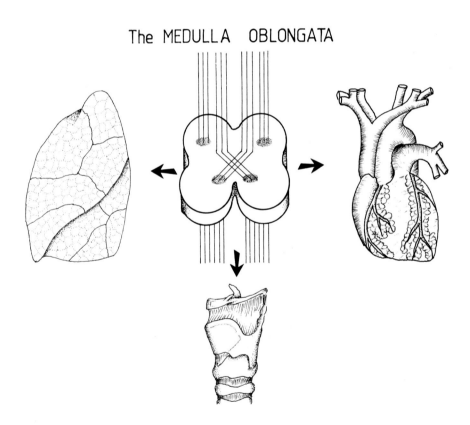

Therefore if there is damage to the base of the skull, as may occur in a head injury resulting from a diving accident, or if a lumbar puncture is done when the intracranial pressure is raised causing herniation of the brain, death will occur.

The majority of motor fibres passing down from the pons to the spinal cord cross over to the opposite side in the medulla oblongata, and tracts of sensory fibres carrying proprioception (position sense from receptors in muscles and tendons) also cross over in this area. It is in the region of the medulla oblongata that the fourth ventricle joins the central canal, and that the eighth, ninth, tenth, eleventh and twelfth cranial nerves arise. Information from the cortex, caudate nucleus and cerebellum is received by the reticular formation in the medulla oblongata, inhibiting the action of the pyramidal system.

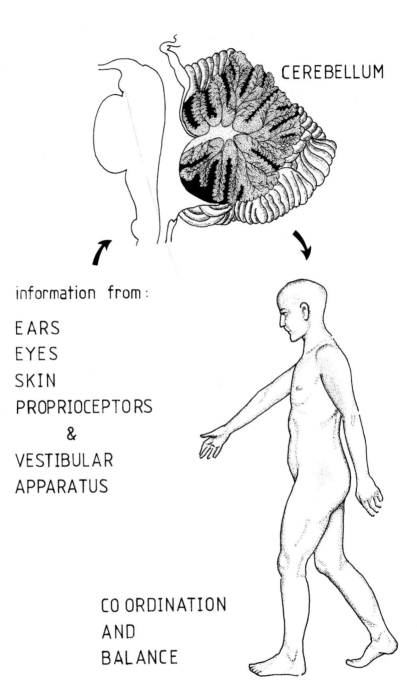

CEREBELLUM

information from:

EARS
EYES
SKIN
PROPRIOCEPTORS
&
VESTIBULAR
APPARATUS

CO ORDINATION
AND
BALANCE

10 The cerebellum

This part of the brain is situated beneath the occipital lobe of the cerebrum and behind the midbrain. The fourth ventricle lies behind it. Separating the cerebellum from the cerebrum is a fold of dura mater called the **tentorium cerebelli.** There are two cerebellar hemispheres joined by a much smaller wormlike structure, the vermis, in the centre. Like the cerebrum, the cerebellum has an outer cortex of grey matter arranged in many fine convolutions, which in section look rather like a tree with its many branches. The inner part consists mainly of white matter or nerve fibres, with a few patches of grey matter. Three bundles of nerve fibres, the **cerebellar peduncles,** join the cerebellum to the medulla, the back of the pons and the midbrain. These are called respectively, the inferior, middle and superior peduncles.

The cerebellum receives information from various parts of the body regarding the latter's position and movement. From the cerebral cortex, information regarding planned movements is sent to the cerebellum before the action occurs. The proprioceptors in the muscles and joints send information regarding their position via the spinal cord. The vestibular apparatus, that is the semicircular canals, the utricle and saccule, send information on the body's position in space and this is supplemented by information from the eyes, ears and skin. This information is received simultaneously, therefore the cerebellum is in a special position to compare it and if necessary modify movement accordingly, via the pyramidal or extrapyramidal tracts, whilst it is in progress. The cerebellum is therefore the centre for co-ordination of muscular movement, particularly that which is learnt. This includes activities such as cycling and typing as well as walking and talking. Because the cerebellum receives information regarding the position of the muscles and tendons it also regulates posture and maintains muscle tone.

CORONAL SECTION

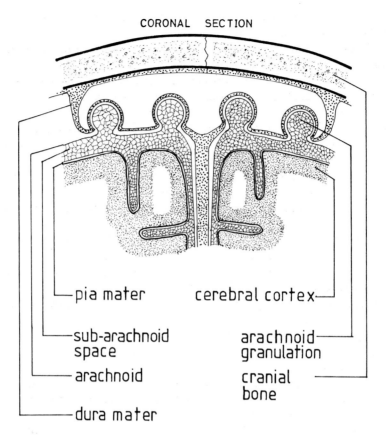

pia mater   cerebral cortex

sub-arachnoid
space   arachnoid
granulation

arachnoid   cranial
bone

dura mater

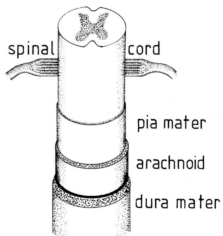

spinal cord

pia mater

arachnoid

dura mater

11 The meninges

The brain and spinal cord are covered by four membranes called collectively the meninges.

The **dura mater,** the outer covering, is a tough fibrous coat consisting of two layers. The outer layer lines the skull, the inner one loosely covering the brain and spinal cord. These two layers are closely adherent, but they separate to form the venous sinuses. The inner layer dips down between the two cerebral hemispheres forming the **falx cerebri.** It also forms a fold separating the cerebral hemispheres from the cerebellum forming the **tentorium cerebelli.** The dura mater is the outer covering of the spinal cord also, but extends beyond the end of the spinal cord to the level of the second sacral vertebra. Between the dura mater and the arachnoid mater is a potential space, the subdural space in which there is a network of blood vessels.

The **arachnoid mater** is an avascular coat also loosely applied to the brain and spinal cord, and closely adherent to the dura mater. It penetrates the dura mater at intervals and forms the **arachnoid villi** or **granulations** which filter cerebrospinal fluid back into the venous system. Between the arachnoid mater and the pia mater is the **subarachnoid space** which contains cerebrospinal fluid. Over the cerebral hemispheres and the major part of the spinal cord this is a very small space, but where the arachnoid mater stretches over the more irregular parts of the brain large spaces are formed which contain cerebrospinal fluid. These are called cisterns. The largest is the **cisterna magna** at the base of the brain between the cerebellum and the medulla oblongata. A cistern of cerebrospinal fluid is also found between the end of the spinal cord and the arachnoid mater.

The **pia mater** is a very delicate vascular membrane containing many small blood vessels supplying the surface of the brain. It adheres closely to the surface of the brain and spinal cord, not only covering the gyri but dipping down into the sulci as well. It dips down into the roof of each ventricle covering small bunches of capillaries which form the choroid plexus and secrete cerebrospinal fluid.

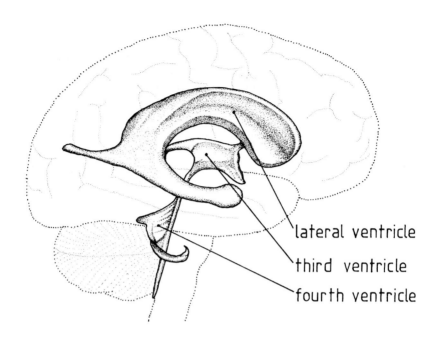

lateral ventricle

third ventricle

fourth ventricle

LATERAL VENTRICLES

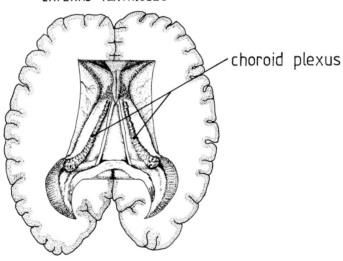

choroid plexus

viewed from above

12   The ventricles

Within the substance of the brain are a series of four cavities of varying sizes called ventricles. The largest of these are the two 'C' shaped **lateral ventricles,** each of which lies deep in the cerebral hemispheres. Connecting the lateral ventricles to the third ventricle are two small openings, the **foramina of Munro.** The **third ventricle** is little more than a slit between the right and left thalami and is connected to the fourth ventricle by a small channel, the aquaduct of Sylvius. The **fourth ventricle** lies behind the pons and medulla oblongata and in front of the cerebellum. It has three small openings, the **foramen of Magendie,** and the two **foramina of Lushka,** which drain into the central canal of the spinal cord and the subarachnoid space respectively. Within the ventricles are tufts of capillaries covered by pia mater which form the **choroid plexus.**

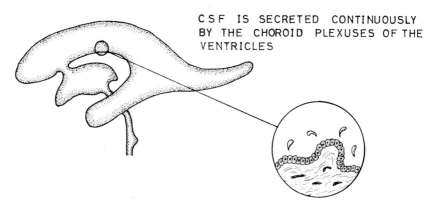

CSF IS SECRETED CONTINUOUSLY
BY THE CHOROID PLEXUSES OF THE
VENTRICLES

CEREBROSPINAL FLUID

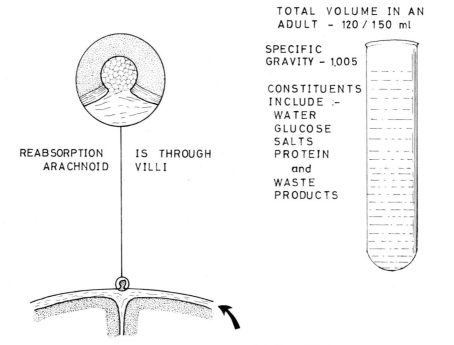

TOTAL VOLUME IN AN
ADULT - 120 / 150 ml

SPECIFIC
GRAVITY - 1,005

CONSTITUENTS
INCLUDE :-
WATER
GLUCOSE
SALTS
PROTEIN
and
WASTE
PRODUCTS

REABSORPTION   IS THROUGH
ARACHNOID   VILLI

CSF   CIRCULATES IN THE
SUBARACHNOID   SPACE

13 Cerebrospinal fluid

In the roof of each of the ventricles are tufts of capillaries covered by pia mater. These are the choroid plexuses and secrete the cerebrospinal fluid. The latter comes directly from the circulatory system and its composition reflects this, being similar to blood plasma but with less protein. From the ventricles the cerebrospinal fluid passes through narrow channels into the subarachnoid space, so bathing the brain and spinal cord. Approximately five hundred millilitres are secreted in twenty-four hours, although there are only one hundred and twenty millilitres in the system at any one time. After circulating around the brain and spinal cord in the subarachnoid space, the cerebrospinal fluid is reabsorbed into the venous sinuses by further clumps of capillaries which penetrate the dura mater. These are called the **arachnoid villi** or **granulations.** Fluid is therefore being constantly secreted and reabsorbed, secretion equalling reabsorption. Blockage in any one of the tiny openings or foramina will interfere with this process and cause an increase in the amount of cerebrospinal fluid, resulting in hydrocephalus in an infant, or raised intracranial pressure in an adult. The normal pressure of cerebrospinal fluid is approximately one hundred millimetres of water. The cerebrospinal fluid acts as a shock-absorber to the nervous system, cushioning it from sudden blows. It also helps to regulate intracranial pressure which may change according to blood flow. Nutrients and waste products probably pass this way also.

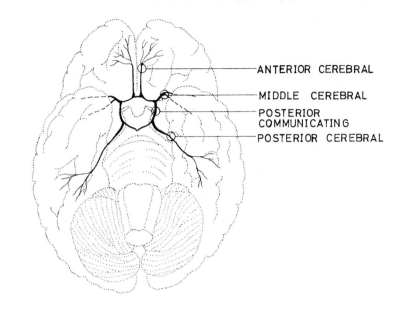

ANTERIOR CEREBRAL

MIDDLE CEREBRAL

POSTERIOR COMMUNICATING

POSTERIOR CEREBRAL

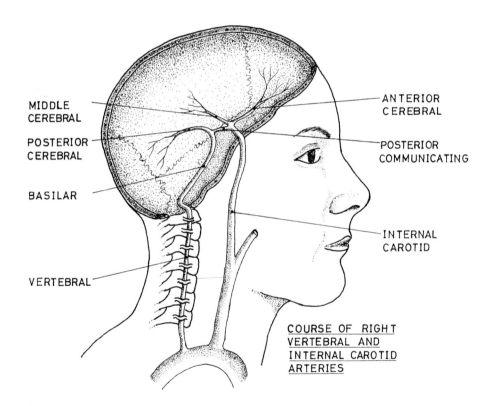

MIDDLE CEREBRAL

POSTERIOR CEREBRAL

BASILAR

VERTEBRAL

ANTERIOR CEREBRAL

POSTERIOR COMMUNICATING

INTERNAL CAROTID

COURSE OF RIGHT VERTEBRAL AND INTERNAL CAROTID ARTERIES

14 Arterial supply of the brain

It is absolutely vital that the brain receives a constant supply of oxygen and glucose via the circulatory system. If it is deprived of either of these substances for more than three to four minutes, as in cardiac arrest or hypoglycaemia, cells will die. Anteriorly the blood supply is from the right and left **internal carotid arteries** which travel up the front of the neck on either side. Posteriorly, the right and left **vertebral arteries** travel up through the cervical vertebrae. The internal carotid arteries each give off two branches, the **anterior cerebral artery** and the **middle cerebral artery**. The vertebral arteries meet to form the short **basilar artery** which gives off two branches, the right and left **posterior cerebral arteries.**

These two separate blood supplies are linked by small blood vessels so completing the **circle of Willis** and ensuring a constant blood supply to the brain. The **posterior communicating arteries** link the posterior cerebral arteries with the middle cerebral arteries. **The anterior communicating artery** links the two anterior cerebral arteries. The anterior cerebral artery supplies the frontal and parietal lobes, the middle cerebral artery supplies the frontal and temporal lobes and also the internal capsule, and the posterior cerebral artery supplies the occipital and temporal lobes. The circle of Willis lies under the base of the brain and in the subarachnoid space.

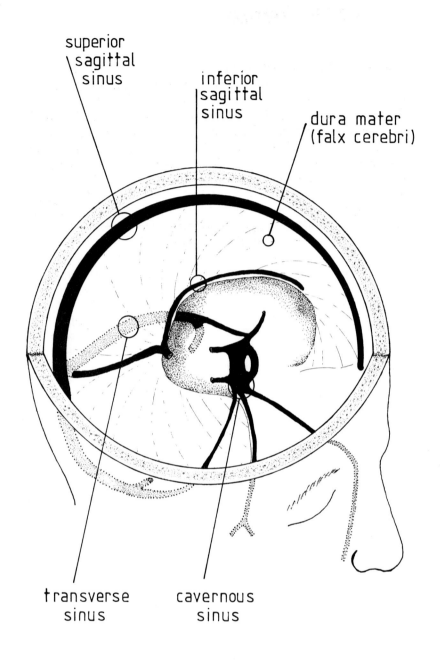

superior
sagittal
sinus

inferior
sagittal
sinus

dura mater
(falx cerebri)

transverse
sinus

cavernous
sinus

DURA MATER and VENOUS SINUSES

15 Venous drainage of the brain

Venous blood is drained by means of venous sinuses which lie between the two layers of the dura mater. Blood drains from the brain into the adjacent venous sinuses. There are many of these linking with each other. The most notable is the **superior sagittal sinus** which travels from the anterior part of the brain along the edge of the falx cerebri to the occipital region. The **cavernous sinuses** lie on either side of the body of the sphenoid bone and the pituitary. The **transverse sinus** travels from the occipital bone past the mastoid bone and eventually into the internal jugular vein. Sepsis and thrombosis may occur in the cavernous sinus from infection of the face, otitis media may cause infective thrombosis of the sagittal and transverse sinuses, and fractures of the skull may damage the internal carotid artery in the cavernous sinus. The venous sinuses eventually drain into the internal jugular vein.

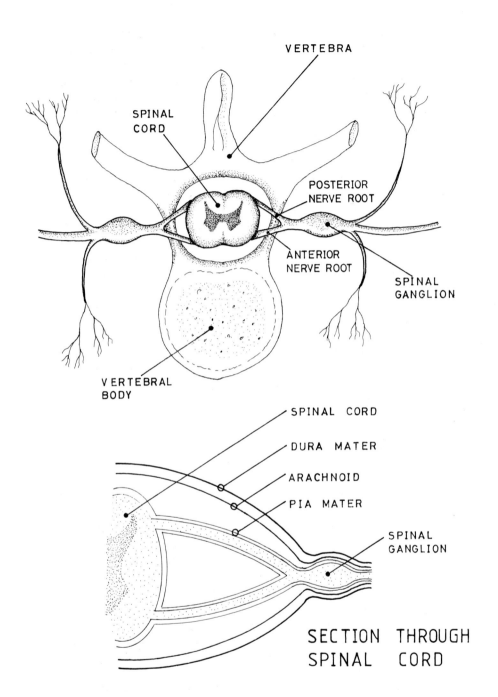

VERTEBRA

SPINAL CORD

POSTERIOR NERVE ROOT

ANTERIOR NERVE ROOT

SPINAL GANGLION

VERTEBRAL BODY

SPINAL CORD

DURA MATER

ARACHNOID

PIA MATER

SPINAL GANGLION

SECTION THROUGH SPINAL CORD

16 The spinal cord

The spinal cord lies in the **vertebral canal** which is formed by the neural arches. It stretches from the foramen magnum in the base of the skull to the level of the second lumbar vertebra, where it is connected to the lower end of the vertebral canal by the fibrous **filum terminale**. Its average length is 45 cm. It is therefore shorter than the vertebral canal. This is because it developed at a slower rate in the fetus. Cylindrical in shape, but slightly flattened posteriorly and anteriorly it measures two centimeters from one side to the other. In the cervical and lumbar regions there is a slight enlargement due to the formation of the nerves into plexuses. Small ligaments along its length hold the spinal cord in position.

Surrounding the spinal cord are the meninges. The pia mater is closely applied to the surface of the spinal cord and also covers the nerve roots. The arachnoid and dura mater extend downwards to the lowest part of the vertebral canal. As cerebrospinal fluid fills the subarachnoid space this forms a cistern at the lower end of the spinal cord and it is here that a lumbar puncture is performed. The arachnoid and dura mater line the vertebral canal and fade out along the spinal nerves.

At regular intervals down the length of the spinal cord the 31 pairs of **spinal nerves** are attached by their posterior and anterior roots, the different sections of the spinal cord being named according to the overlying vertebrae and the spinal nerves leaving it. The cervical region has eight spinal nerves leaving it, the thoracic region twelve, the lumbar region five, the sacral region five, and the coccygeal region one.

The spinal cord is a continuation of the medulla oblongata, and its similarity will be seen in a transverse section. This section shows an outer part of white matter and an inner H-shaped area of grey matter, in the centre of which is the central canal. The white matter consists mainly of nerve fibres which are grouped into ascending and descending tracts. The sensory, or **ascending tracts** fall mainly in the posterior region, whereas the motor or **descending tracts** are mainly in the anterior region. The grey matter contains mainly nerve cells of the motor and association neurones, the sensory cells being found in the ganglia of the posterior root. The upper poles of the 'H' are called the posterior horns, and the lower ones the anterior horns. The cell body of the lower motor neurone is found in the latter. The tiny central canal is a continuation from the fourth ventricle and travels the length of the spinal cord down its centre, containing cerebrospinal fluid.

The function of the spinal cord is to relay information to the brain from the peripheral nerves, to relay information from the brain to the lower motor neurones, and to relay information in and out of the spinal cord.

45

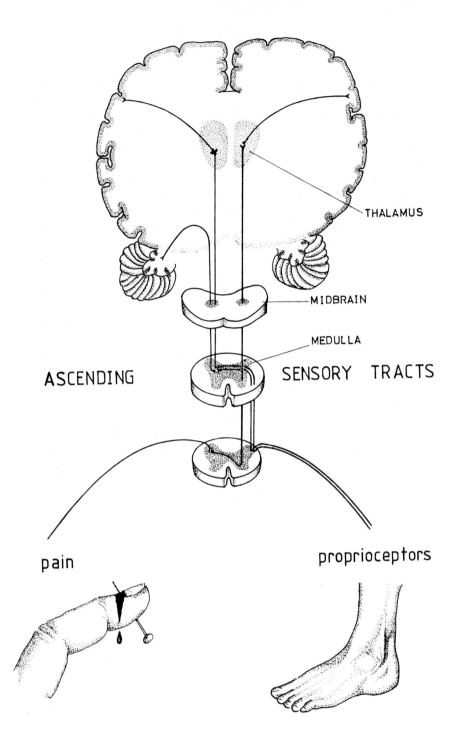

THALAMUS

MIDBRAIN

MEDULLA

ASCENDING   SENSORY   TRACTS

pain

proprioceptors

17   Ascending sensory tracts

The sensations of pain, temperature, and touch are fed into the body from the environment by numerous receptors and nerve endings in the skin. Other sensations regarding position, vibration, discrimination of shape, size, and texture, and accurate localisation of touch, are picked up by receptors called **proprioceptors** in the muscles, tendons, joints, and ligaments. These two groups of sensation are carried by different sensory nerve pathways. Those carrying pain, temperature, and touch from the receptors in the skin enter the spinal cord via the posterior nerve root, cross over and synapse in the cord, and then travel laterally up the opposite side until they reach the thalamus where there is another synapse. The final group of nerve fibres travels to the posterior central gyrus of the cortex via the internal capsule.

Nerve fibres carrying information from the proprioceptors also enter the spinal cord via the posterior root ganglion, but travel posteriorly up the same side of the cord on which they enter, crossing over to the other side of the cord in the medulla oblongata where they synapse. Some branches go to the cerebellum on the same side. From the medulla oblongata fibres travel to the thalamus where there is a further synapse. The final group of fibres goes via the internal capsule to the posterior central gyrus of the cortex, where the information is interpreted.

Both sensory nerve pathways therefore consist of three groups of neurones from the receptor to the brain. As the sensory nerves travel up they will be joined by other groups of nerve fibres entering the spinal cord at higher levels. The first group of neurones in the chain from the receptor to the spinal cord may be part of a reflex arc.

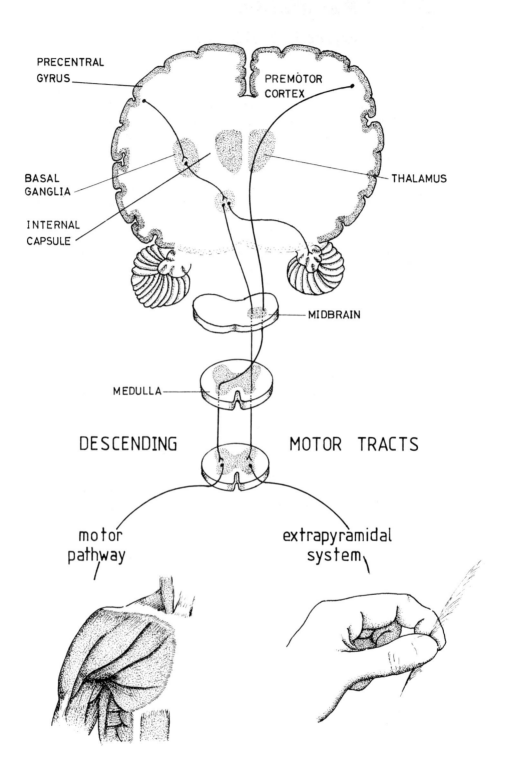

PRECENTRAL GYRUS

PREMOTOR CORTEX

BASAL GANGLIA

INTERNAL CAPSULE

THALAMUS

MIDBRAIN

MEDULLA

DESCENDING MOTOR TRACTS

motor pathway

extrapyramidal system

18 Descending motor tracts

The purpose of the motor pathways is to initiate movement and the descending pathways responsible for initiating voluntary movements form the **pyramidal system**. Motor activity originates in the precentral gyrus of the cortex, situated in front of the central sulcus, where the motor cells are. The fibres from these cells on each side of the brain, converge in the internal capsule. The fanlike arrangement of the fibres is called the **corona radiata**. The fibres then pass down through the brain stem to the medulla oblongata where the majority cross over to the other side, the remainder crossing at a lower level. This crossing of the nerve fibres in the medulla oblongata is called **decussation**. The motor fibres pass down in the anterior part of the spinal cord, synapsing in the anterior horn of the spinal cord with other motor neurones. This second group of neurones travels from the spinal cord to the peripheral muscle. The neurones which originate in the motor cortex and pass down to the spinal cord are called **upper motor neurones**. Some of them may only go as far as the cervical spine, others will go right down to the lumbar spine. The upper motor neurone may therefore vary in length and has no synapse until it reaches the spinal cord. The motor neurones which originate in the anterior horn of the spinal cord, at whatever level this is, are called **lower motor neurones**. These form part of the spinal nerves, and therefore of the peripheral nervous system, and are also involved in spinal reflexes.

Adjacent to the precentral gyrus is the premotor area. Motor fibres coming from the premotor area in the cerebrum, the basal ganglia, and the brainstem, form the **extrapyramidal system** and help to co-ordinate muscular movements and make smooth controlled movements possible. These nerves also travel down the spinal cord and exert their effects on the anterior horn cell, and therefore the lower motor neurone is the final common path.

LIGHT REFLEX

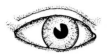 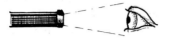 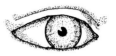

iris muscles contract to make pupil smaller
in bright light

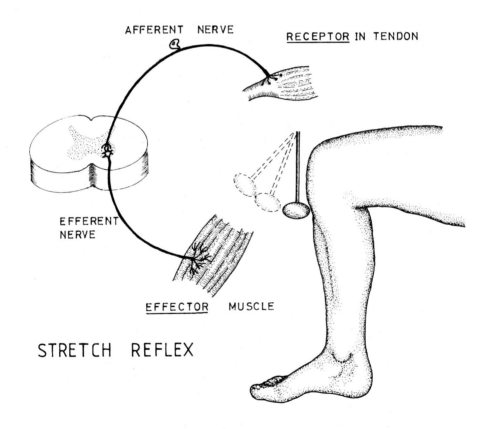

STRETCH REFLEX

19 The reflex arc

Many muscular movements are under the control of the cortex and are a deliberate response to a sensory stimulus. But there are many movements which occur without any conscious decision by the individual. If a puff of wind comes near the eye, a blink occurs, and if someone steps on a drawing pin they smartly withdraw their foot. The information is registered in the cerebrum but the action was not initiated by it. These automatic reactions to a stimulus are called reflexes. Their purpose is to reduce the amount of work the cerebral cortex has to do. They are also rapid, and therefore frequently have a protective function. Some of them are involved in the maintenance of posture and muscle tone.

Spinal reflexes are those which act through the spinal cord. Receptors in the muscles and tendons are stimulated by stretch, so initiating impulses which travel via the sensory neurones of the peripheral nerve to the posterior horn of the spinal cord. Within the spinal cord there may be a direct link with the motor cells in the anterior horn, but more often a connector neurone links the sensory and motor neurones. The impulse then travels out of the spinal cord along the motor neurones to the effector organ, a muscle, causing it to contract. Although these spinal reflexes do not need the brain for their action, sensory information is also sent to the brain via the ascending pathways. Impulses from the brain may be inhibitory, so modifying the action of a reflex.

In order to trigger off a given reflex, stimulation must take place in a specific area; for example the knee jerk is elicited by a sharp tap on the tendon of the quadriceps muscle. When a reflex takes place all the muscles involved in a movement act in a co-ordinated manner. This means that if a muscle contracts, its antagonist relaxes. The greater the stimulus the more effective the action is, so ensuring removal from danger. The speed at which the reflex occurs depends upon the thickness of the nerve fibres, whether the nerve is myelinated or not, and on the number of synapses involved. Thick, myelinated nerves with few synapses will carry impulses most quickly.

Some cranial nerves are also involved in reflexes, such as the **light reflex**, when the pupil of the eye contracts if a light is shone in it. (The pupil of the other eye also contracts and this is termed the consensual light reflex.) Maintenance of posture and muscle tone involves reflexes and there are also superficial reflexes such as the stroking of the skin on the abdomen causing contraction of the underlying muscles. The autonomic nervous system includes reflexes controlling the smooth muscle of organs and blood vessels and the activity of sweat and salivary glands.

Conditioned reflexes are those which occur as a result of training. Certain smells will cause salivation because they are associated with food.

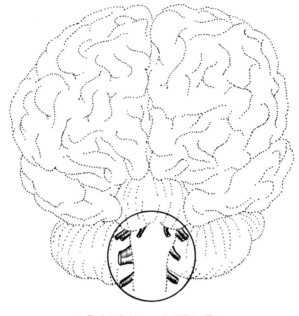

CRANIAL NERVES

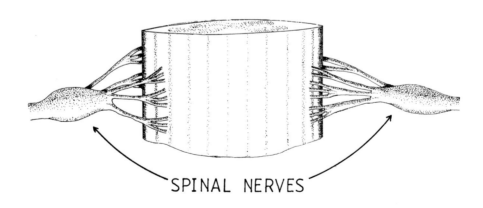

SPINAL NERVES

20 An introduction to the peripheral nervous system

The peripheral nervous system is that part of the nervous system which links the central nervous system with the peripheral parts of the body. It consists of:

The spinal nerves

There are thirty one pairs of spinal nerves which enter and leave the spinal cord, one pair between each pair of vertebrae. They include sensory fibres bringing information from receptor organs in the body to the spinal cord, and motor fibres taking information from the spinal cord to the various parts of the body. The spinal reflexes are therefore part of the peripheral nervous system. As well as motor and sensory information, these nerves also carry fibres from the sympathetic part of the autonomic nervous system. The sacral nerves carry nerve fibres from the parasympathetic system.

The cranial nerves

There are twelve cranial nerves. The nerve cells of these are found in the brain stem and the nerves themselves can be seen on the under surface of the brain. Their connections are mainly within the head and neck, bringing information into the brain from sensory organs such as the eyes and the ears, and sending motor fibres out to muscles and glands. Some of these are completely motor in function, and others sensory, but the majority are mixed. Many of them also carry autonomic nervous system fibres. The vagus nerve (X) has important extracranial branches, supplying organs in the thoracic and abdominal cavities.

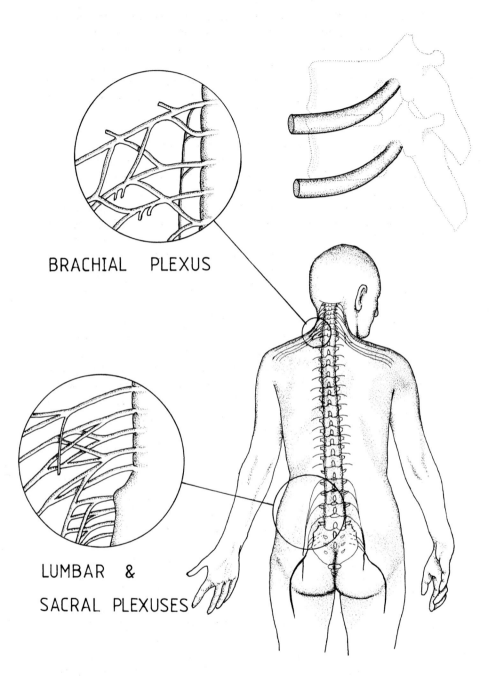

BRACHIAL   PLEXUS

LUMBAR   &
SACRAL PLEXUSES

21 The spinal nerves

Together with the cranial nerves the spinal nerves form the peripheral nervous system. They arise from the vertebral column, and when the fetus is developing leave the cord in a horizontal direction. However as the spinal cord grows, the vertebrae grow faster so that the spinal cord is shorter than the vertebral column. The result is that the spinal nerves come to leave the spinal cord in an oblique manner.

There are 31 pairs of spinal nerves which leave the spinal cord from each side through the openings or foramina between the vertebrae. There are eight pairs of cervical nerves, twelve pairs of thoracic, five pairs of lumbar, five pairs of sacral, and one coccygeal nerve. Apart from the cervical nerves the number of nerves corresponds with the number of vertebrae. There is an extra cervical one because there is one pair of cervical nerves leaving between the skull and the first cervical vertebra, and also one between the seventh cervical and the first thoracic vertebra.

As the spinal nerves leave the spinal cord some of them group together to form plexuses, where the nerve fibres recombine to follow the most direct route. The first four cervical nerves form the **cervical plexus**, supplying the head and neck. The remainder of the cervical nerves and the first thoracic form the **brachial plexus**, supplying the arms. The **lumbar plexus** consists of the first four lumbar nerves which supply the front of the leg. The last two lumbar nerves and the first three sacral nerves form the **sacral plexus** supplying the buttocks and the back of the legs. The thoracic nerves do not form a plexus, but just encircle the chest in bands supplying the adjacent areas of skin and muscle. Individual spinal nerves receive sensation from a specific area of skin which is called a **dermatome**.

Each spinal nerve is attached to the spinal cord by a posterior root with a ganglion and an anterior root. The **posterior root** consists of sensory nerves coming from the receptors in the skin and muscle, their cell bodies being in the ganglion on the posterior root. The **anterior root** consists of motor nerves taking information from the spinal cord to the muscles. These two roots combine to form the spinal nerve, which is therefore a mixed nerve containing both sensory and motor fibres. As they leave the spinal cord, the spinal nerves divide into a small posterior branch which supplies the skin and muscle of the back, and a larger anterior branch which supplies the skin and muscle of the front and sides of the trunk and also of the limbs. It can be seen that the spinal nerves form the major part of a spinal reflex arc, and include the lower motor neurone.

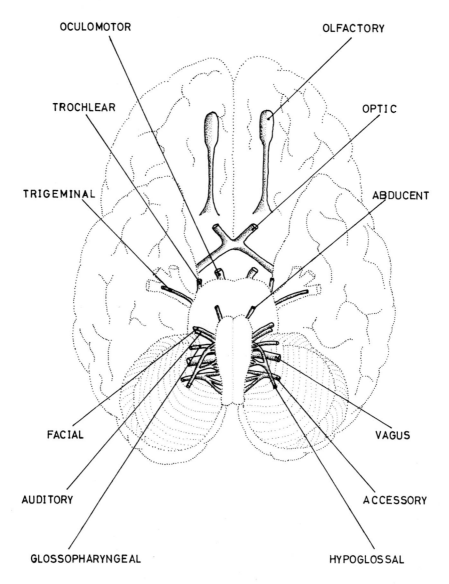

OCULOMOTOR

OLFACTORY

TROCHLEAR

OPTIC

TRIGEMINAL

ABDUCENT

FACIAL

VAGUS

AUDITORY

ACCESSORY

GLOSSOPHARYNGEAL

HYPOGLOSSAL

CRANIAL NERVES

22 The cranial nerves

There are twelve pairs of cranial nerves all of which arise at different levels in the brain stem except the olfactory (I) and the optic (II).

I	Olfactory	Sensory	Smell – from receptors in the nose
II	Optic	Sensory	Sight – from the retina of the eye
III	Oculomotor	Motor Autonomic	Movement of the eyes Size of pupil
IV	Trochlear	Motor	Movement of the eyes
V	Trigeminal	Sensory Motor	Face Muscles of chewing
VI	Abducent	Motor	Movement of eyes
VII	Facial	Sensory Motor Autonomic	Taste Facial expression Salivary glands
VIII	Auditory	Sensory	Cochlear branch – hearing Vestibular branch – balance
IX	Glosso-pharyngeal	Sensory Motor Autonomic	Taste Pharynx Parotid gland
X	Vagus	Sensory Motor Autonomic	Palate, pharynx vocal cords Palate, pharynx, vocal cords All the thoracic and abdominal organs
XI	Spinal Accessory	Motor	Muscles of neck
XII	Hypoglossal	Motor	Movement of tongue

BRACHIAL PLEXUS

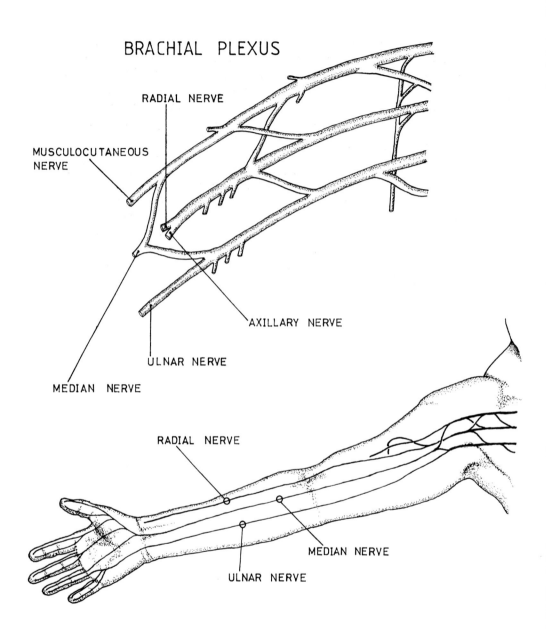

RADIAL NERVE

MUSCULOCUTANEOUS
NERVE

AXILLARY NERVE

ULNAR NERVE

MEDIAN NERVE

RADIAL NERVE

MEDIAN NERVE

ULNAR NERVE

23 The nerves
of the upper limb

The anterior branches of the spinal nerves in the lower cervical region (C5–T1) leave the spinal cord at the level of the lower part of the neck. They link up together forming the **brachial plexus**, which travels via the axilla to supply the arm. Any pressure in the axilla, as from crutches, or the abnormal movement which may occur with bad lifting techniques in a paralysed patient, can damage the nerves and so interfere with the function of the arm.

There are five main nerves leaving the brachial plexus, which with their branches supply the muscles and skin of the arms and hand. These are the **musculocutaneous nerve** supplying the muscles at the front of the arm as well as the skin of the lower outer arm, the **median nerve** supplying the flexor muscles and the skin of the palm and the two outer fingers, the **ulnar nerve** supplying the small muscles of the hand, the **axillary nerve** supplying the shoulder muscles and the overlying skin, and the **radial nerve** supplying the extensor muscles and the skin of part of the arm and hand.

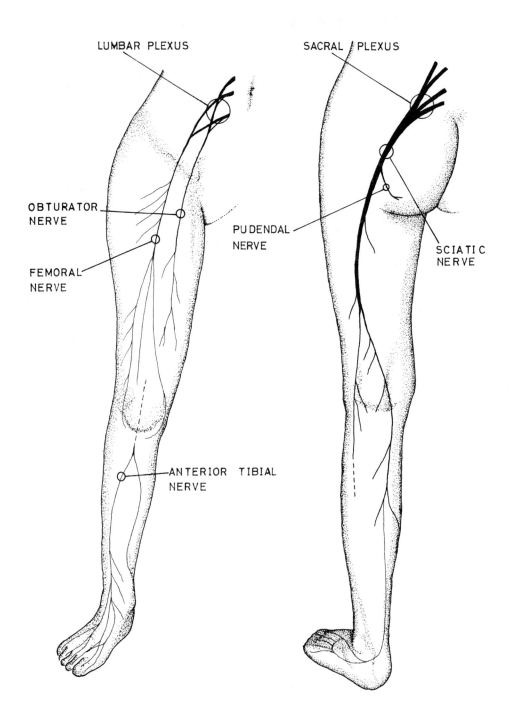

LUMBAR PLEXUS

SACRAL PLEXUS

OBTURATOR
NERVE

PUDENDAL
NERVE

FEMORAL
NERVE

SCIATIC
NERVE

ANTERIOR TIBIAL
NERVE

24 The nerves of the lower limb

The fourth lumbar and the sacral spinal nerves form the **sacral plexus** which passes in front of the sacrum but then travels through the obturator foramen of the pelvis to the back. As it passes posteriorly it becomes narrower to form the sciatic nerve. Branches are given off to form the gluteal nerve supplying the muscles of the buttocks, and the pudendal nerve supplying the anal and urethral sphincters and external genitalia. The **sciatic nerve** is the largest nerve in the body. It lies behind the ischium and runs straight down the centre of the posterior part of the leg giving off branches to the muscles of the legs and feet.

Damage can occur to the sciatic nerve if an intramuscular injection is given in an incorrect position in the buttock. A prolapsed intravertebral disc may press on its roots, giving rise to a typical distribution of pain and wasting.

The obturator nerve arises from the lumbar nerves passing through the obturator foramen to divide into an anterior and posterior branch which supply the thigh and the knee.

The other major nerve supplying the leg is the **femoral nerve** arising from the **lumbar plexus**. The femoral nerve with its branches supplies the front of the leg.

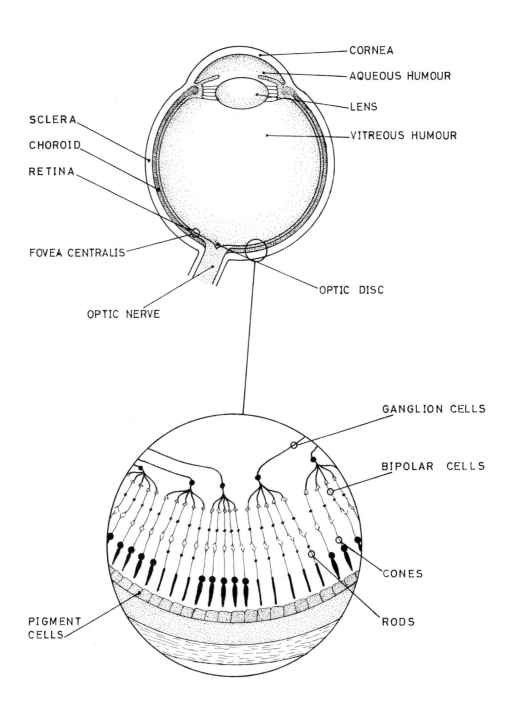

CORNEA

AQUEOUS HUMOUR

LENS

VITREOUS HUMOUR

SCLERA

CHOROID

RETINA

FOVEA CENTRALIS

OPTIC DISC

OPTIC NERVE

GANGLION CELLS

BIPOLAR CELLS

CONES

PIGMENT CELLS

RODS

25 Sight

The **retina**, the inner layer of the eye, is composed of specialised receptor cells called **rods** and **cones** which are sensitive to light. The rods are spread across the retina but are absent in the fovea centralis. They are sensitive to low levels of light but are not sensitive to colour. The cones are concentrated in the centre of the retina and particularly in the **fovea centralis**. They require a higher level of light to stimulate them and are sensitive to colour. In the fovea centralis the layers of nerve cells are pushed to each side so that light falls directly on the cones, ensuring maximum vision. Each rod or cone is linked to a bipolar cell neurone which in turn connects with a ganglion cell neurone, the axons of which form the optic nerve.

The rods and cones contain pigments which are broken down chemically by the various wavelengths of light. In the rods the pigment is called **visual purple** (rhodopsin). Light breaks it down into substances which initiate nerve impulses. In darkness the rhodopsin is regenerated again if there is sufficient vitamin A available. It takes a short period of time therefore to become 'dark adapted' while the rhodopsin is being regenerated.

The cones are thought to be of three different types, each one sensitive to a different wavelength of light, i.e. red, green and blue. Stimulation of different combinations to different intensities is thought to account for the range of colours we can see. The retinal layer next to the choroid coat consists of pigment cells which prevent light spreading from one receptor to another.

The light waves enter each eye through the **cornea**, **lens**, and **vitreous humour**, each of which causes them to be bent slightly and therefore directed onto a small area of the retina at the back of the eye. These light waves then cause the chemical changes already described to take place in the rods and cones. This initiates a nerve impulse in the connecting neurones. The impulse passes through a series of neurones which cross the retina and converge to form the **optic nerve**, leaving the eye posteriorly. This point is known as the 'blind spot' or **optic disc**, which can be seen with an ophthalmoscope.

The images from each visual field fall slightly out of true with each other so giving stereoscopic vision. Light from the outer or temporal fields of each eye falls on the inner or nasal area of the retina. It travels along each optic nerve to the **optic chiasma** where it crosses over to the other side and travels via the optic tracts and the optic radiations to the occipital part of the brain. Light from the nasal fields of each eye falls on the outer temporal area of the retina and travels along the outer part of the optic nerve but does not cross to the other side in the optic chiasma, instead it links up with the brain on the same side. The image received by the brain is inverted.

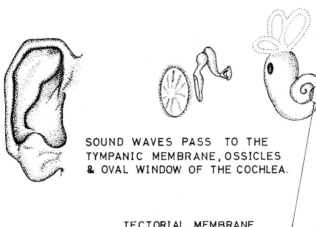

SOUND WAVES PASS TO THE
TYMPANIC MEMBRANE, OSSICLES
& OVAL WINDOW OF THE COCHLEA.

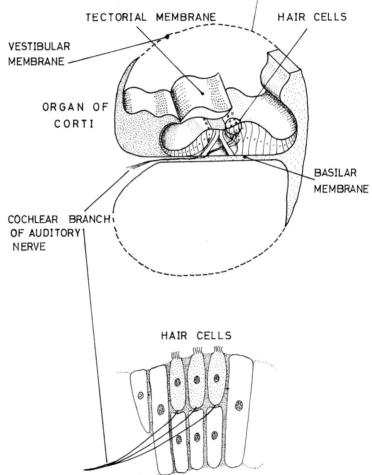

TECTORIAL MEMBRANE

HAIR CELLS

VESTIBULAR
MEMBRANE

ORGAN OF
CORTI

BASILAR
MEMBRANE

COCHLEAR BRANCH
OF AUDITORY
NERVE

HAIR CELLS

26 Hearing

The receptors of hearing are found in the **cochlea** of the inner ear. The cochlea is a spiral tube, divided into three channels along its length by two membranes. They are the **basilar and vestibular membranes**. The basilar membrane is wider at one end than the other. In the central canal and along the surface of the basilar membrane is the **organ of Corti**. This consists of **hair cells** whose processes are capped by the **tectorial membrane**. These hair cells connect with the cochlear branch of the auditory nerve. It is thought that different frequencies of sound cause different parts of the basilar membrane to vibrate so stimulating different sections of the organ of Corti.

Sound waves are picked up by the pinna of the ear and pass through the external auditory meatus causing the tympanic membrane to vibrate. Three small bones (ossicles), the **malleus**, **incus**, and **stapes**, are arranged in such a way that they magnify the movement. Because the malleus is in contact with the tympanic membrane it also moves, transmitting the vibration to the incus and stapes in turn. The foot of the stapes is resting on the membrane of the **oval window** of the cochlea, and it therefore moves the **perilymph**, the fluid inside. This vibrates the basilar membrane and causes the tectorial membrane to distort the hair processes of the hair cells, so initiating a nerve impulse. The nerve impulse passes along the cochlear branch of the auditory nerve. After synapsing at the junction of the pons and the medulla oblongata, crossing over to the other side, and synapsing again in the brain, the nerve fibres finally reach the auditory area in the temporal lobe of the cerebral cortex where the information is interpreted. The **round window** in the cochlea allows the pressure to equalize.

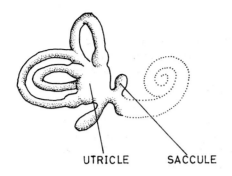

UTRICLE   SACCULE

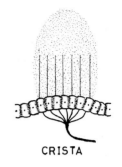

CRISTA

otoliths

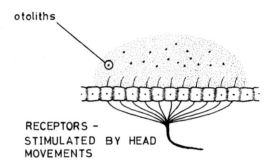

RECEPTORS -
STIMULATED BY HEAD
MOVEMENTS

vestibular apparatus
of BALANCE

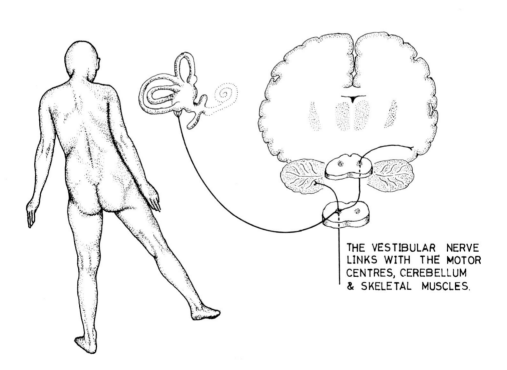

THE VESTIBULAR NERVE
LINKS WITH THE MOTOR
CENTRES, CEREBELLUM
& SKELETAL MUSCLES.

27 Balance

Hearing and balance are very closely connected. The vestibular apparatus consists of the three **semicircular canals**, the **utricle** and **saccule**. Each of the semicircular canals is in three different planes and contain the fluid **endolymph**. At the ends of the canals are enlarged areas called the ampullae, which contain the receptor organs. In each of these are groups of hair cells connected to a jelly-like mass. These are the **cristae**. Starting or stopping movements of the head cause movement of the endolymph within the semicircular canals, so moving the cristae and initiating nerve impulses. These impulses travel along the vestibular branch of the auditory nerve to the cerebral cortex, branches also going to the cerebellum where the information is co-ordinated. Immediately beneath the semicircular canals, where they join together, is the utricle and continuous from this is the saccule. These also contain hair cells with hair processes connected to a jellylike mass. However in the latter there are tiny calcium deposits called **otoliths** which are sensitive to gravity. Changes in the position of the head stimulate these nerve endings, the impulses also passing along the vestibular branch of the auditory nerve to the cerebral cortex.

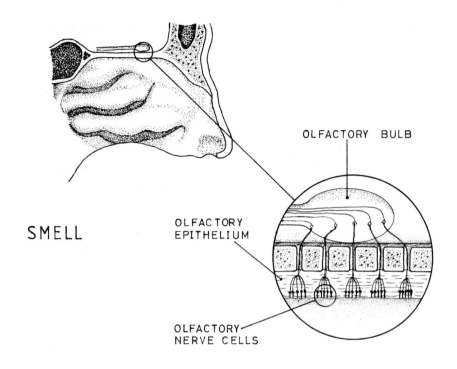

OLFACTORY BULB

OLFACTORY
EPITHELIUM

SMELL

OLFACTORY
NERVE CELLS

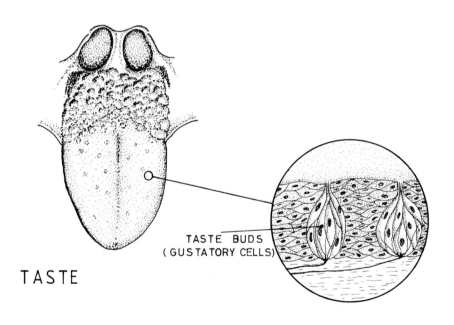

TASTE BUDS
(GUSTATORY CELLS)

TASTE

28 Smell and taste

The receptors for smell are situated in a very small area of the mucous membrane in the upper part of the nose. The processes from these receptors pass up through tiny openings in the thin plate of bone immediately above and end in the **olfactory bulb**. The latter lies immediately below the frontal lobe of the cerebrum. Nerve fibres go from the olfactory bulb to special centres in the cerebrum. A smell in the form of a gas enters the nasal passages and is dissolved in the secretions so forming a chemical solution. This chemical stimulates the receptors which initiate nerve impulses in the olfactory nerve. These impulses travel along the olfactory nerve to the special areas in the cerebrum where they are interpreted.

Many substances which appear to stimulate the sensation of taste are in fact stimulating the organ of smell. This is why any condition interfering with the ability to smell, such as the common cold, will diminish the sense of taste also. Remaining in the presence of a particular smell for even a short time causes the receptors to adapt, and therefore the smell is no longer apparent. If a fresh smell is introduced the receptors are immediately sensitive. The sense of smell may be destroyed (anosmia) in certain types of head injury, or frontal lobe tumours, or it may become more acute if the adrenal cortex is underactive.

The receptors for taste are found primarily on the surface of the tongue although the palate and the pharynx are also sensitive. The surface of the tongue is covered with tiny projections or papillae with tiny pits between them. In these pits are the **taste buds** or receptors. These taste buds appear to be sensitive to four different sensations, salt, sweet, sour and bitter. Each of which is found in a different area of the tongue. The front portion is sensitive to sweet and salt, the sides to sourness and the posterior to bitterness. The receptors in the front two-thirds of the tongue link with a branch of the facial nerve (VII) whereas those in the posterior third link with the glossopharyngeal nerve (IX). These nerves synapse in the medulla oblongata and again in the thalamus, the final nerve travelling to an area in the parietal lobe of the cerebrum.

Flavours from food chewed in the mouth are dissolved in the saliva to form a chemical substance which stimulates the receptors in the tongue. This initiates nerve impulses in the facial and glossopharyngeal nerves which travel to the medulla oblongata. From there the impulses travel to the thalamus and then onto the cerebrum where the taste is interpreted in the light of previous experiences.

TOUCH

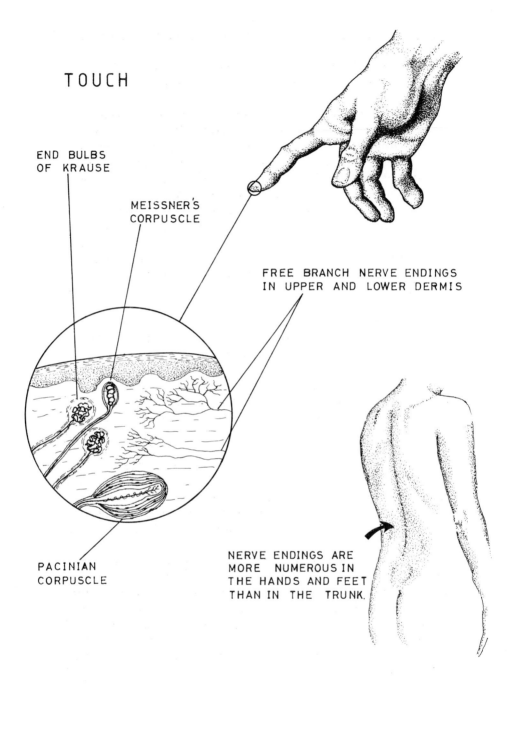

END BULBS
OF KRAUSE

MEISSNER'S
CORPUSCLE

FREE BRANCH NERVE ENDINGS
IN UPPER AND LOWER DERMIS

PACINIAN
CORPUSCLE

NERVE ENDINGS ARE
MORE NUMEROUS IN
THE HANDS AND FEET
THAN IN THE TRUNK.

29   Touch

The skin not only has the function of temperature control and acting as a protective covering for the body, but is also a large sensory organ. Within it are a great many receptors which are sensitive to the five sensations of touch, pressure, pain, warmth and cold.

The receptors for touch appear to be of two different types, bare nerve endings and **Meissner's corpuscles**. The latter are coiled nerve endings containing little discs which are encapsulated. They are found in the fingers and other very sensitive areas. The **Pacinian corpuscles** are found under the skin and more deeply in certain parts of the body. They are also encapsulated and when looked at under a microscope have a layered appearance like an onion. It is considered that they are pressure receptors being stimulated by compression of the skin. Pain receptors are thought to be bare nerve endings. Cold and heat are possibly picked up by **Ruffini** and **Krause endings**, or possibly bare nerve endings. Bare nerve endings are also found at the base of the hair follicle and are stimulated by the movement of the hair even if the skin itself has not been touched. It therefore seems that the different receptors help to differentiate the type of stimulus to some extent, although the brain is responsible for interpreting the information.

The intensity of a sensation, that is whether a stimulus is felt as merely warm or very hot, depends upon the rate of the impulses. The greater the stimulus the greater the rate of impulses per second. It is possible to localise sensation remarkably accurately; the hand is particularly sensitive and can discriminate between two points very close together, the trunk less so. This is related to the amount of representation of the different parts of the brain. If a stimulus continues over a long period of time adaptation takes place and the individual ceases to be aware of it unless a change occurs or one is directed to think about it. For example one soon forgets the pressure of a chair when sitting or one's clothes unless reminded of them.

All these nerve endings join up with one another to form a network of nerves which travel to the spinal cord and enter via the posterior root. Therefore together with the nerves from the proprioceptors they form the sensory part of the reflex arc, linking up with the motor nerves. They also send branches up the spinal cord to the brain (*see* 17–Ascending Sensory Tracts). It is in the cerebral cortex behind the central sulcus that the information is received and interpreted.

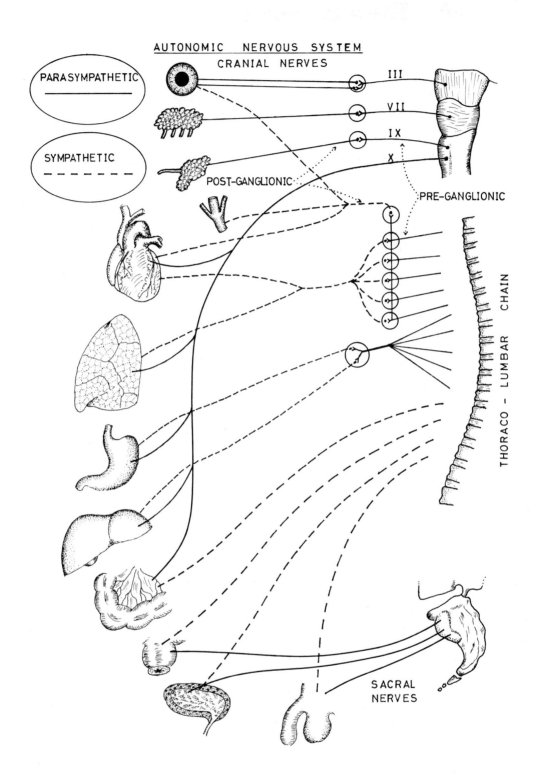

AUTONOMIC NERVOUS SYSTEM

CRANIAL NERVES

PARASYMPATHETIC

SYMPATHETIC

III

VII

IX

X

POST-GANGLIONIC

PRE-GANGLIONIC

THORACO - LUMBAR CHAIN

SACRAL NERVES

30 The autonomic nervous system

The autonomic nervous system is in control of all those functions of the body that take place automatically, such as the secretions of glands and the constriction of smooth muscle in blood vessels and organs.

The hypothalamus has a controlling influence over it, as well as over the endocrine system, and therefore the two systems have a close relationship. The autonomic nerves originate in the lower centres of the brain leaving the central nervous system via the cranial, thoraco-lumbar and sacral nerves. The autonomic system is divided into two branches, the sympathetic and the parasympathetic, each being complementary to the other.

The sympathetic nervous system

The neurones of the sympathetic nervous system leave the spinal cord with the thoracic spinal nerves and the first three lumbar spinal nerves, they are therefore also called the **thoraco-lumbar chain**. At this point the nerves are myelinated and are called the preganglionic fibres. Outside the spinal cord the preganglionic fibres synapse with other nerves in a ganglion. These are called postganglionic fibres and are usually not myelinated. The ganglia of the sympathetic nerves form a chain down either side of the vertebral column and this is called the sympathetic chain. Some of these ganglia are grouped together into plexuses. The most important of these being the cardiac plexus and the solar (coeliac) plexus in the abdomen.

The sympathetic nervous system is stimulated in situations of stress such as the 'fright, fight, and flight' response. Those organs not required for this type of situation have their blood supply and activity reduced, whereas those needed have an increased blood supply. The blood supply is increased to the heart and voluntary muscles by vasodilation, the heart rate is increased, the bronchioles relax, the pupils dilate, and hair stands on end. At the same time the medulla of the adrenals secretes more adrenaline, the liver mobilises liver glycogen and the sweat glands are active. These are all activities necessary to flight. At the same time other activities are decreased. The blood supply to the gut and genitalia is decreased and the stomach, small intestines, and colon relax and become less active, secreting less, so decreasing digestive processes and sexual activity. The bladder wall relaxes, and the sphincters of the bladder and anus constrict inhibiting defaecation and micturition. The secretions of the salivary glands are diminished. These are all activities which are not necessary in the flight situation. The

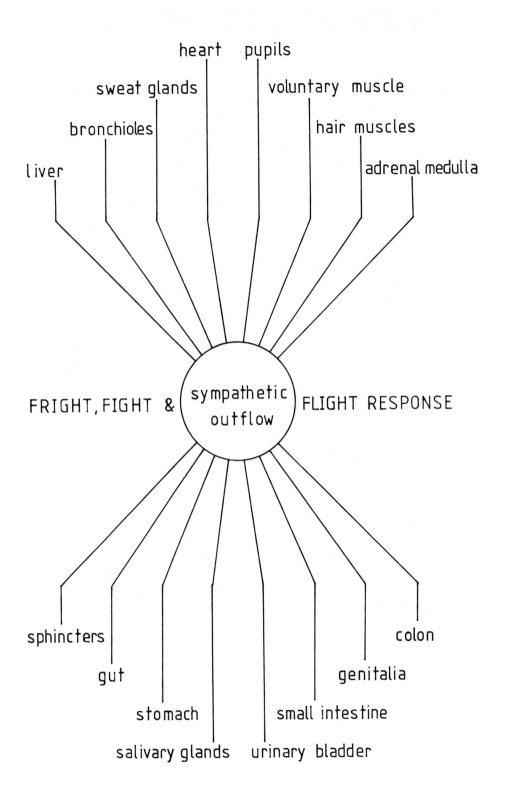

sympathetic system is also involved in heat regulation, by increasing heat loss from the body by dilating surface vessels and sweating.

The parasympathetic nervous system

The neurones of the parasympathetic nervous system leave the central nervous system with the third, seventh, ninth and tenth cranial nerves, and the second and third sacral nerves. This branch is also called the **craniosacral** outflow. In this case the postganglionic fibres are close to the organ being supplied, and not the vertebral column.

The parasympathetic becomes active when the individual is in the relaxed state, and tends to work in the opposite manner to the sympathetic. Each branch which leaves with a cranial nerve has a specific effect. The oculomotor (III) constricts the pupil and controls accomodation for near vision. The facial (VII) stimulates the production of tears by the lacrimal duct, and with the glossopharyngeal (IX), saliva from the salivary glands. The vagus (X) supplies a large number of organs. It slows the heart, constricts the coronary blood vessels and bronchial muscles and stimulates the secretion of the gastric glands and the peristaltic contraction of the gut and the gall bladder. Those branches leaving with the sacral nerves contract the urinary bladder, relax the anal and urethral sphincters and cause vasodilatation in the genitalia. The parasympathetic is therefore active in the digestive processes, micturition and defaecation, and sexual activities, all of which are best suited to a state of relaxation.

Chemical transmitter substances

At the end of all nerve fibres there is a chemical transmitter substance released. In the autonomic system there are two such substances, noradrenaline and acetylcholine. Noradrenaline is released at the end of all the postganglionic nerve fibres of the sympathetic branch (except those supplying the sweat glands). These are called **adrenergic** fibres. Acetylcholine is released at the end of the preganglionic fibres of both the sympathetic and parasympathetic nervous system, and the post ganglionic fibres of the parasympathetic system, and the sweat glands. These are called **cholinergic** fibres.

SENSORY NERVE PATHWAYS

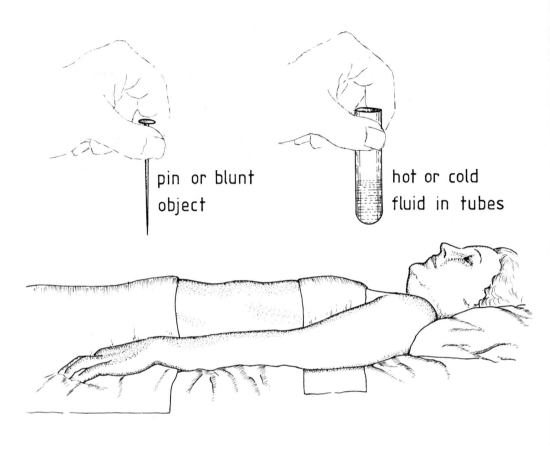

pin or blunt object

hot or cold fluid in tubes

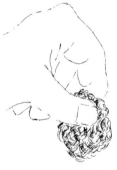

cotton wool

areas of anaesthesia can be mapped out - the patient responds to particular sensations e.g. pain or touch

31 Neurological examination

The purpose of the doctor's neurological examination is to test the functioning of the various nerve pathways. It includes an assessment of cerebral and cerebellar function and motor and sensory nerve pathways.

Preparation of the patient

The patient's co-operation will be required with many of the tests and therefore it is very important that he knows what is required of him. Much of the examination may appear irrelevant, therefore a full explanation will be given as to what is going to be done and why. The patient is asked to undress down to his underclothes and lie on a couch covered with a blanket. Dressing gown and slippers should be available.

Cerebral function

The patient's mental state is assessed by noting whether he responds normally to questions or is disorientated. The doctor will listen for any slurring of his speech or difficulty in remembering words. The patient may be asked to do a simple calculation such as subtracting seven from one hundred and continuing to subtract seven from the remainder. Memory will be tested on recent events.

Sensory nerve pathways

The patient is asked to close his eyes and say when he feels the particular sensation. Areas of anaesthesia will be mapped out using a skin pencil.

Pain: The point of a pin is used to test the surface of the skin for superficial pain. Deeper pain requires pressure with a blunt object.

Temperature: Glass or metal tubes containing hot and cold water can be used for this test.

Touch: The surface of the skin is touched slightly with cotton wool.

Vibration: A tuning fork is vibrated and then placed on the ankle bone and at the wrist.

Motor nerve pathways

The limbs are inspected for any wasting, comparing the left with the right. A tape measure may be used for a more accurate assessment. The patient is then asked to hold out his arms with the fingers splayed out. Any tremor or weakness will be apparent. The power

CRANIAL NERVES

Olfactory
patient asked to smell
substances through
each nostril

Optic
retina examined
with ophthalmoscope

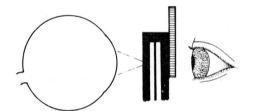

Auditory
ears are inspected
and tested for
deafness

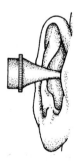

of each group of muscles is tested by trying to overcome them, the patient resisting by pushing in the opposite direction. The grip of each hand will also be tested. All the important reflexes will be tested with a patella hammer including those at the elbow, knee and ankle. The plantar reflex will be demonstrated by stroking the inner aspect of the sole of the foot, the toes normally curling down. If they go upwards and the toes fan out (Babinski's sign), this indicates damage to the upper motor neurone, although this is the normal response in a baby. Abdominal reflexes occur in response to stroking the abdomen, the muscles contracting. Reflexes require both sensory and motor pathways to be intact and will therefore reveal damage to either. Although the upper motor neurone is not necessary for a functioning reflex it does have a modifying effect upon it, and if damaged will result in exaggerated reflexes. Lesions of the cerebellum also influence the action of the reflex causing the limb to continue swinging.

Cranial nerves

I *Olfactory:* One nostril is blocked and the patient is asked to smell small bottles containing substances such as oil of cloves, peppermint or lavender. The other nostril is then tested.

II *Optic:* The retina is examined with an ophthalmascope for **papilloedema** (swelling of the optic disc) and damage to the retinal vessels. Visual acuity is tested with a Snellen's chart, the patient being asked to identify the letters with each eye in turn. The visual fields are examined by asking the patient to close one eye and look straight ahead with the other, the doctor gradually introducing a white object from the side, and the patient indicates when he can see it.

III *Oculomotor*	The patient is asked to look up, down and to either side in order to check the ability to move the eyes.
IV *Trochlear* VI *Abducens*	Any continuous abnormal jerking of the eyes (**nystagmus**) is noted, and the reaction of the pupils to light, as well as any drooping of the lids or retraction.

V *Trigeminal:* Cotton wool and a pin are used to note any loss of sensation over the face. A wisp of cotton wool used to touch the cornea will cause automatic blinking (the corneal reflex).

VIII *Auditory:* The ears are inspected with an auroscope to ensure no wax is interfering with hearing. By means of whispering, and using a watch and a tuning fork, the doctor will test the level of hearing. The tuning fork is vibrated and held near the ear being tested. When it can no longer be heard it is then placed over the mastoid bone, where, in conductive deafness it will be heard more

PROPRIOCEPTION

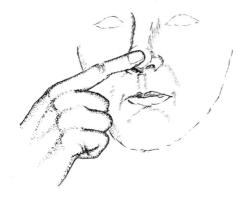

touch the nose
with the finger

stand with the
eyes closed
(Romberg's test)

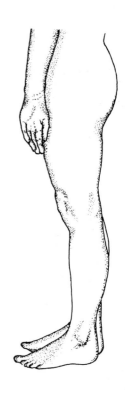

clearly. The tuning fork can also be placed in the centre of the forehead to discriminate between conductive and nerve deafness. The sound is louder in the good ear in nerve deafness, and in the affected ear if conduction is the problem.

IX *Glossopharyngeal:* The tongue is blotted and a solution of either sweet, sour, bitter or salt is dropped onto the tongue. A more reliable method is to apply an electrical stimulus.

X *Vagus:* The patient is asked to make certain sounds, and the movement of the soft palate is observed. His ability to swallow fluids and cough normally is noted, and also if there is any change in the voice.

XI *Spinal accessory:* The patient is asked to shrug his shoulders.

XII *Hypoglossal:* The patient is asked to put out his tongue and any wasting or abnormal movement is noted.

Proprioception

This includes information coming from within the body from tendons, muscles and joints. The patient is asked to close his eyes and his big toe is moved by the doctor in different directions. The patient then indicates the direction he believes the toe is being moved in, by moving his hand in the same direction. He is then asked to stand with his eyes closed, and the nurse must be ready to catch him if he falls (**Romberg's test**). This will happen in tabes dorsalis where the sensory nerve pathways are damaged. He is then asked to walk with one foot in front of the other in a straight line, so that the gait may be observed. Co-ordination is tested by asking the patient to close his eyes and bring the finger of his outstretched hand to touch his nose; he also does it quickly with his eyes open. Another test for co-ordination is to ask the patient to run the heel of one foot down the shin of the other leg.

Cerebellar function

Tests of co-ordination, gait and the response of the reflexes will all give information as to the efficient functioning of the cerebellum. The patient may also be asked to hold a familiar object such as keys or a coin in his hand with his eyes closed to see if he can recognise it.

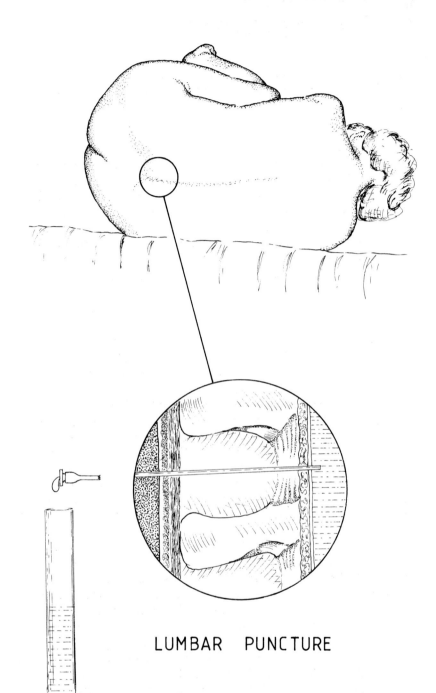

LUMBAR PUNCTURE

32 Neurological investigations

Initially the doctor will do a thorough neurological examination, but if there are positive findings he may need to do further investigations.

Lumbar puncture

The lumbar puncture is one of the first investigations likely to be performed. It is done to take a small specimen of cerebrospinal fluid to examine it for the presence of blood, micro-organisms, and changes in its composition. It may also be used to introduce substances to enable X-rays to be taken of the subarachnoid space around the spinal cord and brain, and the ventricles. Drugs and anaesthetics may be introduced this way (intrathecal). A lumbar puncture is not done if there is raised intracranial pressure, because herniation of the brain will occur (coning).

It should be explained to the patient that a local anaesthetic will be used and therefore they will only feel this and not the actual procedure. They will also be told that after the procedure they may have a headache but this is usually relieved by lying down and analgesics will be given if necessary. The patient is normally placed in an exaggerated left lateral position, the knees well up and the head tucked down, so that the back is rounded. The back will lie parallel to the edge of the bed and the patient will have a pillow under the head. If the patient is obese, fracture boards are placed under the mattress to prevent lateral curving of the spine. Care should be taken that the patient is not pressing on the abdomen. This position will ensure that the spinal processes open up and make it easier for the doctor to introduce the needle. This is an aseptic technique and every care must be taken to prevent the introduction of infection. After anaesthetising and cleansing the area the doctor will introduce the lumbar puncture needle between the third and fourth lumbar vertebrae, the spinal cord ending at the end of the first lumbar vertebra. The pressure will be measured by a manometer. At this point the doctor may ask the nurse to press on the jugular vein in the neck, which will normally cause a rise in the pressure (Queckenstedt's sign). Absence of this rise indicates spinal block. He will then wish to take two or three specimens of cerebrospinal fluid. The nurse will hold the specimen bottle under the end of the needle to catch the drops of fluid. The bottles must be carefully labelled in the order in which they were taken. After the doctor has removed the needle the puncture wound is sealed. The patient will be asked to lie flat for at least six hours and maybe up to 24 hours. Lying on his abdomen or raising the foot of the bed may be necessary if the headache persists. Fluids should be encouraged.

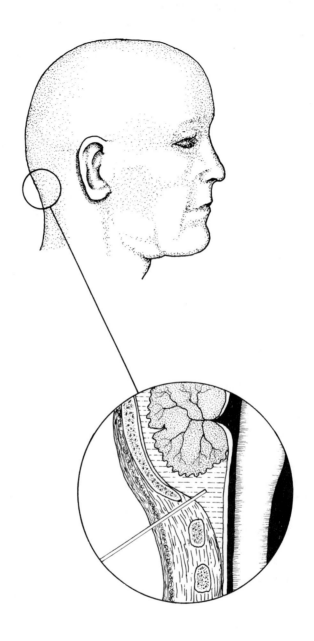

CISTERNAL   PUNCTURE

Cisternal puncture

This is a puncture into the cisterna magna beneath the occiput. It is done if there is a spinal block, and sometimes for myelography. In this case the back of the neck and the occipital region up to the occipital protuberance are shaved. Usually the patient is sat up with the head bent forward, although it can be done with the patient lying on his side. The procedure is the same as for lumbar puncture, although sometimes the pressure is so low that a syringe is needed to withdraw the fluid.

Myelography

This investigation is done in the X-ray department in order to locate pressure on the spinal cord which might occur from a tumour or prolapsed intravertebral disc. Because the substance used is iodine-based a skin test should be done to check for allergy. Following a lumbar puncture, radio-opaque oil (Myodil) is injected into the subarachnoid space. The patient is then tilted so that the Myodil flows in the direction required and the radiologist screens the patient. He is then able to mark the spot where the pressure occurs. Myodil does not normally cause any ill-effects but does take a considerable time to be absorbed. Therefore Metrizamide, a water soluble substance which is quickly absorbed, is often used instead. If the latter is used the patient will be sat up afterwards and should not bend the head forward, otherwise the dye will reach the brain and may cause epilepsy in some patients.

Air encephalography

This investigation is also done in the X-ray department, but in a sitting position. The procedure is sometimes carried out under a general anaesthetic, in which case the relevant preparation must be given. Even if it is done under a local anaesthetic, analgesics and anti-emetics are given beforehand. A lumbar puncture is performed, air being introduced through the needle. The air will rise to the ventricles and so it will be possible to take X-rays in which the brain stem and the cerebral hemispheres are outlined and also to show the ventricles.

Ventriculography

This procedure is normally carried out in theatre when raised intracranial pressure prevents a lumbar puncture being done. The head is shaved and the patient prepared as for an operation. The patient is starved even if it is not intended to carry out the procedure under a general anaesthetic, because it may be necessary to anaesthetise the patient during the procedure. Air is introduced directly into the ventricles through burr holes.

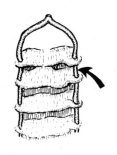

vertebral
artery

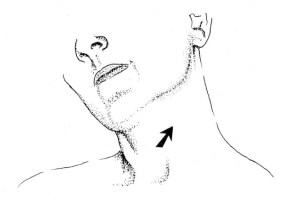

carotid   artery

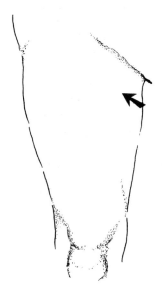

ANGIOGRAPHY

femoral
artery

the   radio-opaque   solution
is   introduced   into   the
vertebral   or carotid artery
or through a fine catheter
passed   into   the   femoral
artery.

Angiography

This is another X-ray investigation, in which the radio-opaque substance Urografin is introduced into the carotid or vertebral arteries. The dye may be injected directly into the artery, or a fine catheter passed under X-ray control into the femoral artery in the groin and from there passed into the carotid or vertebral arteries. This X-ray causes an unpleasant burning sensation in the face and behind the eyes which the patient must be warned about. He should also be told of the importance of keeping still. After the procedure he should be watched for bleeding from the site, and if it occurs pressure should be applied. Two hourly neurological observations will be taken.

Electroencephalogram (EEG)

This involves the application of electrodes to the head in order to measure electrical currents in the brain. Abnormal activity may sometimes be demonstrated in patients with a brain tumour or epilepsy. Negative findings do not necessarily mean that the brain is normal.

Brain scan

A radioisotopic substance is injected into a vein from where it travels through the circulation to the brain. If a cerebral tumour, abscess or vascular disorder is present this will cause an increased uptake of the substance so producing a positive brain scan.

Computerised axial tomography (CAT Scan)

This is a method of X-raying the patient in such a way that the X-rays give pictures at various depths. A computer is used to measure the amount of X-ray absorption and a very accurate picture can be built up. Because this does not require the injection of any substances it is a harmless procedure. It does require the patient to remain still for twenty minutes and therefore an unco-operative patient may require sedation.

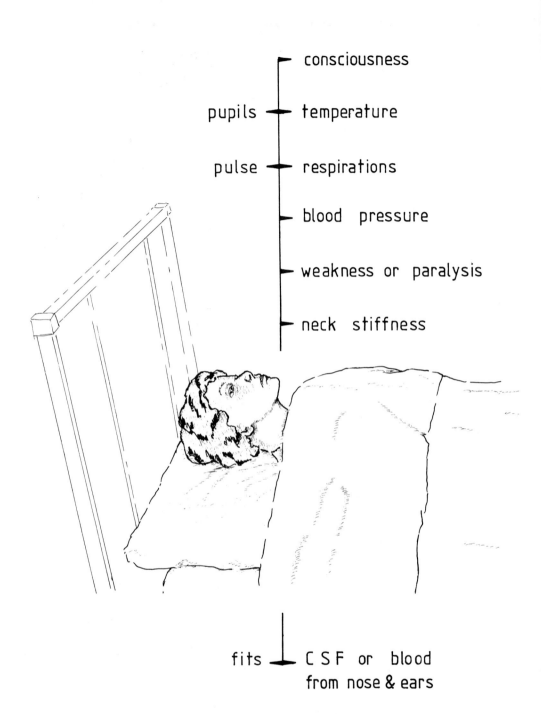

consciousness

pupils — temperature

pulse — respirations

blood pressure

weakness or paralysis

neck stiffness

fits — C S F or blood
from nose & ears

33 Neurological observations

Early assessment is vital in order to set a baseline, as prompt recognition of changes can prevent irreversible brain damage and death.

Level of consciousness

A brief description of the exact response of the patient is better than vague terms such as 'semiconscious'. The following is one method of recording.

Unconscious: The patient fails to respond to painful stimuli, which may be applied in various ways such as gripping the Achilles tendon in the heel firmly.

Unconscious but responding to painful stimuli: This may be by withdrawal of the part from the stimulus or by making sounds. The stimulus should be applied to each side in turn, and a note made if there is any difference, which may indicate paralysis. Flexion or extension of the limbs when responding is also noted.

Conscious but not fully orientated: If the eyes are closed the nurse should speak to the patient by name to see if they are opened in response. Direct commands may then be given, and a note made as to the speed of response. When it is possible to talk to the patient he can be asked his name and address and other simple questions. Any disorientation or confusion will gradually show itself. Any period of amnesia should be recorded, particularly if the patient has had a head injury.

Fully conscious and able to talk coherently: It is important to notice any *changes* in the level of consciousness and to report these promptly.

Pupils

These are examined to see that they are equal and of normal size. Enlargement of one indicates haemorrhage or herniation of the brain on that side. The pupils should react briskly to a strong light with a narrow beam by constricting as the beam of light falls on each of them in turn. The other pupil should constrict at the same time (consensual reflex). The pupil does not react in a blind eye.

Blood pressure, temperature, pulse and respiration: In raised intracranial pressure the blood pressure rises in an effort to maintain the circulation to the brain, and the pulse becomes slow and bounding. At a later stage the respirations become slower and irregular. Damage in the region of the hypothalamus will cause changes in the temperature, usually hyperpyrexia.

Fits and other observations: Appropriate observations should be made of any fits occurring. The nose and ears should be checked for any leakage of cerebrospinal fluid or blood.

Maintenance of the airway

Skin care

Care of the mouth

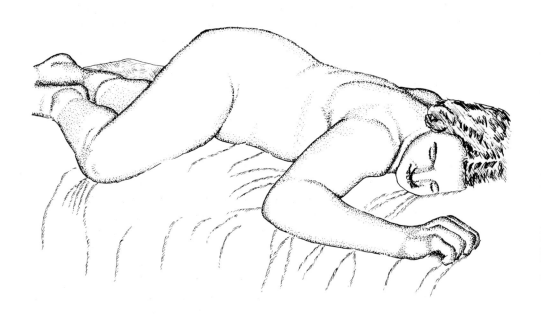

Care of the eyes

Care of the bladder

Care of the bowels

34 Nursing care of the unconscious patient

The unconscious patient is unable to maintain the normal activities of the body without assistance. The aim is to maintain life support and to prevent any complications arising.

Maintenance of the airway

It is essential to check that there is no foreign body such as false teeth blocking the airway. The patient will be positioned in such a way as to ensure that the tongue does not obstruct the airway, usually in the semi-prone position. Suction will be necessary to clear secretions. In some patients an airway will be inserted, or even an endotracheal tube or tracheostomy if respirations are inadequate. The quality of the respirations should be monitored carefully as they may be too shallow to be adequate. On the other hand there may be hyperventilation due to acidosis, which can be corrected by intravenous therapy. Turning two hourly will help to prevent the development of respiratory infection, and it is important to recognise the early signs of this so that prompt treatment may be initiated.

Skin care

Because the patient is not moving spontaneously he is at risk of developing pressure sores unless vigorous preventive measures are taken. He should be turned two hourly, each position change being recorded on a turning chart. A large cell ripple-bed will help to vary pressure. When the patient is on his side care will need to be taken to prevent one leg pressing on the other. A protected pillow or foam wedge can be placed between the two legs. Badly placed urinals or bed cradles can press against the patient causing a sore. Tubifoam over heels or elbows helps to protect these. Cleanliness of the skin is necessary not only to prevent pressure sores but to maintain the health of the skin and provide protection from infection. This is particularly so where two surfaces meet such as in the axillae or under the breasts. If the hands become clenched they should be gently opened and washed. The feet will accumulate hard dry skin and may need to be oiled.

Care of the mouth

Even though the patient is not eating, secretions will accummulate in the mouth and pharynx. It is essential to keep the mouth moist and clean to prevent infection. A good light must be used to look in the mouth and check that it is clean. If there is paralysis, special attention will have to be paid to that side. Swabs must be held firmly by clipped forceps, and should not be too moist.

91

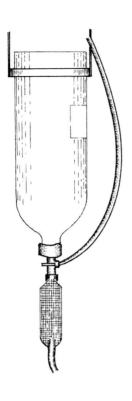

NUTRITION & FLUIDS
initially intravenous
then naso-gastric

ACCURATE OBSERVATIONS

fluid balance
neurological
blood pressure
temperature
pulse
respirations

record
with care

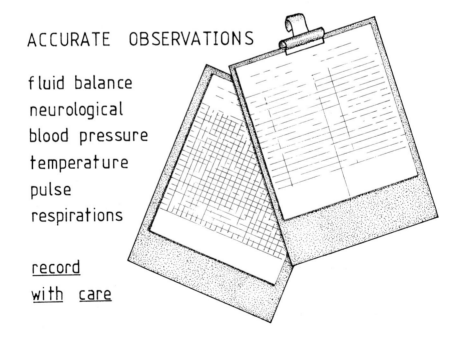

Care of the eyes

These are kept closed with a light pad and tape. They are cleansed two hourly with sterile normal saline, and kept lubricated with light liquid paraffin. Any evidence of infection such as a sticky eye will require swabs to be taken, and appropriate treatment will be prescribed by the doctor.

Care of the bladder

Depending on the cause of the unconsciousness, the patient may either be incontinent or have retention with overflow, and will therefore require catheterisation. Catheter toilet will be carried out regularly, and aseptic changing of the urinary drainage bag daily. If the patient remains unconscious for any length of time, the catheter is changed weekly unless it is a special type of catheter. With men, incontinence appliances or a urinal placed in position may be found to be more appropriate. Observations for urinary tract infection will be necessary.

Nutrition and fluids

Initially the fluid intake may be controlled by the intravenous route. After the first 24 hours a nasogastric tube will be inserted. The fluid diet must be well balanced with an adequate amount of calories, protein and vitamins, as well as fluid and electrolytes. Good nutrition is essential to prevent tissue breakdown.

Prevention of deformity

Care in positioning the limbs is vital to prevent damage leading to permanent paralysis. The patient should never be dragged up the bed by the arms because this may result in damage to the brachial plexus and to the skin. Passive movements will be carried out by the physiotherapist and supplemented by the nurses when attending to the patient, in order to prevent spasticity and deformity of the limbs. A cradle will help to prevent foot drop.

Observations

A raised temperature will usually indicate infection which could be present in the lungs or bladder although hyperpyrexia may suggest damage in the region of the hypothalamus. Measures will have to be taken to reduce the temperature by tepid sponging, fans, etc. The fluid loss will also need to be replaced. The blood pressure will be monitored particularly if there is the possibility of raised intracranial pressure, when it will rise, and neurological observations will be necessary. The fluid balance chart will be necessary to monitor both urinary output and fluid intake.

Psychological care

Although the unconscious patient is unable to respond, this does not mean that he is unaware of what is happening to him or what people are saying. Therefore the nurse will be careful what she says in his presence, as well as talking to him and explaining what she is going to do before carrying out a procedure.

93

HEMIPLEGIA

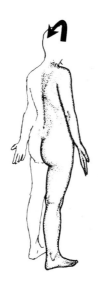

one side of the body is
affected – may be caused
by a cerebral vascular
accident on the opposite
side to the paralysis

PARAPLEGIA

paralysis from the waist
down due to damage to
the spinal cord at a low
level e.g. spina bifida

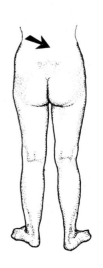

TETRAPLEGIA

all four limbs and possibly
breathing are affected due
to damage to the spinal
cord at a high level
e.g. poliomyelitis

35 The paralysed patient

PATHOLOGY

A patient may develop paralysis in any part of his body due to trauma, disease processes or congenital abnormalities. The paralysis has a defined pattern according to which nerves are affected.

Hemiplegia, hemiparesis
One side of the body is affected, with weakness or complete paralysis. Cerebrovascular accident is the most common cause, the lesion being in the brain on the opposite side to the paralysis (an upper motor neurone lesion). If the dominant hemisphere is affected then speech will also be involved. Other space-occupying lesions including tumours and large aneurysms may also have the same effect.

Paraplegia
Paralysis occurs from the waist down as a result of damage to the spinal cord at a low level. Meningomyelocele, a developmental abnormality, trauma, and diseases such as multiple sclerosis or polio may all result in this type of paralysis. A paraplegia interferes with bladder and bowel function.

Tetraplegia
All four limbs are paralysed and because the lesion is the result of damage to the spinal cord at a high level the respiratory muscles may also be affected. Road traffic accidents, sporting accidents, such as diving in insufficient water, or a disease such as polio, may cause it.

Monoplegia
Paralysis of one limb may occur through damage to the nerves supplying that limb, or may sometimes be due to hysteria.

NURSING CARE PLAN

Many paralysed patients, such as those with a cerebrovascular accident, may be unconscious in the initial stages and this, togther with some of the aspects of caring for a patient with a hemiplegia, is covered in Chapter 37. The care of a patient with a tetraplegia is very specialised and is not covered. The nursing care is aimed at helping the patient to be as independent as possible. At first a great deal of help will be needed even to do very basic activities. The patient's attitude towards his condition, and the degree of

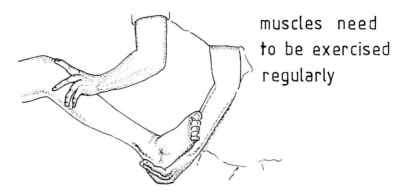

muscles need
to be exercised
regularly

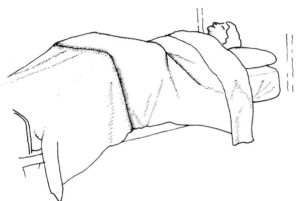

cradles relieve the
pressure on paralysed
limbs

help the patient to
become as independent
as possible

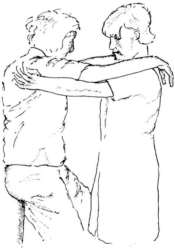

determination to make the most of what he has, will make the difference between success and failure. There will be many times when he will become depressed and will need the encouragement of those helping him. The hemiplegic may ignore the paralysed half of his body and will have to be constantly made aware of its existence.

Prevention of pressure sores

The paralysed patient is at great risk of developing pressure sores because the nerve supply to the skin is diminished, and added to this the patient is unable to move. He may therefore not be aware that damage is occurring,and sores may quickly develop. Where the patient is unable to relieve the pressure by lifting himself, the nurse must do it for him. Particular care must be taken when removing bedpans or placing urinals. Aids for the prevention of sores will be necessary, but even more important is a nourishing diet. The areas at risk must be carefully inspected for any redness and where it occurs immediate action taken. Pressure sores may also occur due to calipers if these are used to strengthen the legs, and they must therefore be put on with care and the legs inspected for signs of pressure when they are removed.

Management of bladder and bowel

Initially the patient will probably be incontinent although retention of urine may occur with a paraplegia. The patient with a hemiplegia may eventually be trained to go to the toilet regularly so preventing an accident. The main difficulties will be mobility and the management of clothing. Hand rails and raised toilet seats may help, and the clothing must be suitable. A patient with paraplegia may be able to express the bladder regularly so preventing leakage. If the bladder is not fully emptied infection is liable to occur. Suppositories or disposable enemas may be used on a regular basis.

Mobility

Whether the paralysis is on one side or involves the lower half of the body there will be problems of balancing. The physiotherapist will therefore do exercises to help the patient compensate, and therefore not fall over so easily. Muscles that are not paralysed have to be strengthened because they will be called upon to do extra work. This is particularly true of the arms in a patient with paraplegia. The paralysed limbs will also be put through a range of passive movements initially, and as movement returns the patient will be able to carry out assisted movements using slings and pulleys. Eventually the patient may be able to move his limbs actively, but may need strengthening exercises.

Because stability is affected, aids will be used to provide this. The patient with a hemiplegia will find a tripod more stable than a walking-stick although he may eventually progress to this. The

recovery from
paralysis includes
balance, stability
and walking

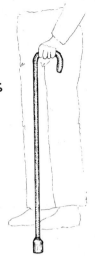

a firm walking stick
may be sufficient

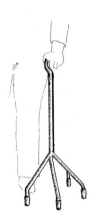

a tripod may be
more beneficial
for the patient
recovering from
hemiplegia

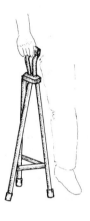

early walking aids
include parallel
bars

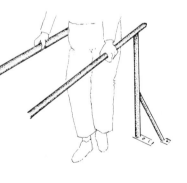

patient with a paraplegia may remain confined to a wheel-chair, or occasionally may begin to walk again with the aid of calipers and a walking frame. Variety is important in maintaining the patient's interest in his exercises, and if there is a useful end product this may provide shorter term goals. For the patient confined to a wheel-chair, sports such as archery, table tennis and swimming help to develop important muscles. Large weaving on an upright frame can be used to encourage the patient with hemiplegia to use his affected arm, even though he may have to lift it up initially with his good one. Care must be taken when lifting and positioning paralysed patients because they are unable to recognise when abnormal stretching is taking place.

Daily living activities

Complete independence means patients returning home and managing for themselves, and preparation must be made for this. The patient must learn to dress himself, and wash and feed himself. The occupational therapist will teach him how to dress in stages, but the nurse may be present when he is putting this into practice, and on no account should she hurry the patient. Clothing will need to be adapted to make it easier to put the garments on, and gadgets may be used to enable the patient to put shoes and stockings on.

The patient with hemiplegia will also have difficulties in feeding himself. Food that can be picked up in the hand is easier to handle and does not require such a steady hand. Special rims fitted to the plate, non slip mats, and cutlery with specially designed handles, all help the patient to become independent. He should be sat up to a table, and have his false teeth in and his glasses on, rather than be left slumped down in bed. Some food will have to be cut up, and food that is difficult to manage avoided. If the face is paralysed on one side he will be encouraged to put food into the non paralysed side and drink afterwards. Gradually other household activities will be introduced, and any helpful gadgets.

MULTIPLE SCLEROSIS

patchy degeneration of the myelin
sheath covering
the nerve

possible causative
factors include:-
linolenic acid deficiency.
vulnerability to virus
infections.
auto-immunity.
trauma.

the myelin sheath
regenerates and function
is restored.
repeated episodes form scar tissue
and complete loss of function in
that particular pathway

36 Multiple sclerosis

PATHOLOGY

Multiple sclerosis is a condition affecting the central nervous system, in which there is patchy degeneration of the myelin sheath covering the nervous tissue. Although the cause is unknown, certain facts are available which have given rise to various theories. Patients suffering from multiple sclerosis are deficient in the fatty acid linolenic acid which may have a protective function. Whether the deficiency is due to the type of diet or not is not known. It is thought that neurones in these people may be vulnerable to a viral infection which is more likely to occur if they grow up in a temperate climate. It is thought by some to be due to an auto-immune response. Minor physical trauma appears to act as a trigger.

Patches of inflammation develop on the myelin sheath, temporarily interfering with its function of transmitting impulses. However, the myelin sheath is regenerated and function restored. After repeated episodes scar tissue forms and there is complete loss of function in that particular pathway. The disease attacks particular nerves such as the optic nerve, cerebellum and the pyramidal tracts. It may attack one or both sides. Multiple sclerosis is a condition primarily affecting those between the ages of twenty and forty, occurring slightly more in women than in men.

Initially there may be an isolated incident such as loss of vision, tripping or dropping things, and patients may easily tire. As these incidents may occur without warning there is a fear of what may happen next, and therefore increasing dependence on others. The pattern varies with each patient, but typically there will be a series of relapses and remissions of varying lengths of time. Gradually the symptoms become more severe and the remissions shorter. Eventually there may be a paraplegia with incontinence and spasticity of the limbs. Urinary infection, pneumonia and pressure sores may eventually cause death.

NURSING ASSESSMENT

Nursing care problems in multiple sclerosis are discussed here in relation to the female patient, in view of the increased incidence in females already referred to. This patient is likely to be of an age when she is married with young children, and the income from her employment may be an essential part of the family finances. The type of work her husband does and the hours he works will influence how great a part he plays in the home life. Do they run a car? If so this will increase mobility. Do they live in a bungalow

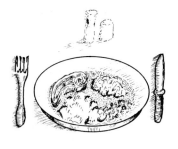

is the patient well
nourished ? - problems :-
dysphagia or nausea.
the effort is tiring.
intention tremor.
facial weakness.

paralysis with impaired
sensation can result in
pressure sores particularly
to the sacral area and
the heels

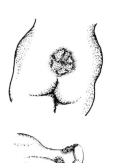

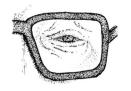

sight may be affected :-
blurred vision.
double vision.
loss of sight.

which can be easily adapted or a flat several stories high? How old are the children? Do they attend nursery school or school? Do the parents of the patient live nearby? How near to the hospital do her relatives live? Can they visit easily?

Her religion may be a very vital part of her life, therefore the name and address of the minister of her church should be noted, and whether she wishes the hospital chaplain to visit her.

General appearance

The nurse will note how well nourished the patient is, and if she is thin or emaciated the cause must be sought. It may be that her diet has been inadequate due to dysphagia or nausea. On the other hand, although she may have had a good appetite the effort of eating may have been so tiring that she could only eat small amounts at one time. Intention tremor, shaking of the hand when moved, may be very frustrating when trying to feed oneself. Facial weakness, spasticity of the hands and a tendency to tire easily are all likely to lead to a reduced diet. In the early stages of the disease the diet may deteriorate simply because she is afraid to go out alone, or due to depression. Conversely, the latter may lead to obesity. The nurse must find out tactfully how much help she needs in feeding and if she has any special equipment at home.

Condition of the skin

If there is any paralysis, and particularly if sensation is impaired, pressure sores will develop unless special care is taken. The sacral area and the heels are the most vulnerable. Diminished sensation may mean that the patient is unaware of a sore until it has become sizeable. Any spasticity of the limbs, which frequently develops in the later stages, will increase the likelihood of sores developing, as will a poor nutrition.

Mental state

The patient's appearance will give some indication of this. Is she making the most of herself, with make-up and hair well kept, or is there a general unkemptness about her appearance. Depression, apathy, anxiety or anger may be her reaction to having the condition, although mood changes are frequently associated with multiple sclerosis. In the early stages irritability is often present, and euphoria may result in unrealistic expectations of the future. It will be necessary to find out from the doctor or her relatives how much she has been told and how she has reacted so far. If she knows her diagnosis then she may have decided to adopt the 'sick role'. It will be useful to find out what her hobbies are and if the ability to do these has been interfered with in any way. For example, she may find it difficult to sew because her fingers fumble and are less sensitive. How well does she sleep? Early waking suggests depression.

urinary problems include:-
urgency.
retention with overflow.
incontinence.
urinary infection

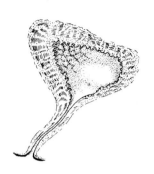

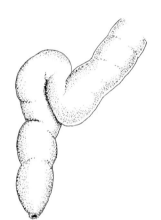

constipation.
spurious diarrhoea.
incontinence of faeces.
may have occurred

take careful note of :-
prescribed drugs.
self medication.

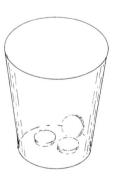

Mobility

The patient may be admitted at any stage of the disease and will have different problems accordingly. In the early stages mobility may be reduced more because of the fear of falling, or the possibility of another sudden attack of blindness, than by real limitations in movement. Blindness will inhibit the patient from moving in an unfamiliar environment, and dizzy spells, blurred vision, and general tiredness may all be factors which cause the patient to be less mobile than usual. Later, paraplegia may be present. But even with a paraplegia there will be varying degrees of dependence. Can she get in and out of a wheelchair with or without help? Does she need help with dressing? Has she been able to have a bath? These are all things the nurse needs to know.

Excretion

There may be urgency, retention with overflow, or complete incontinence, depending upon the stage of the disease. Frequency, a burning sensation on passing urine, or a raised temperature, may indicate an urinary infection. Constipation, spurious diarrhoea, or incontinence of faeces may be present and the method of control before admission must be discovered.

Special senses

There may be blurring of vision, double vision or complete loss of sight. It is necessary to know how long the patient has had these disturbances of vision because this will have influenced how well she has adapted. Occasionally there is deafness. Speech is often staccato, becoming slow and deliberate, or slurred and therefore less easy to understand.

Observations

A raised temperature may be present due to infection in the lungs or bladder, and will therefore be monitored carefully. Any drugs she has brought with her, or any self-medication, will be noted.

NURSING CARE PLAN

The patient with multiple sclerosis has a slowly progressive disease. The nursing care plan will therefore be evaluated regularly and adjusted to take into consideration new problems.

Care of the skin

As the patient develops paralysis and becomes less able to care for herself, so the role of the nurse changes. In the initial stages the patient will be taught how to relieve pressure on the buttocks by raising herself in the chair at least two hourly. Once confined to bed she will be turned by the nurses two hourly, although a 'monkey pole' may enable her to lift herself in bed, and a sheepskin or ripple

105

proteins
vitamins —→ a nourishing diet
fluids
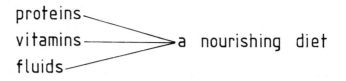

weigh the patient weekly

avoid fatigue.
passive exercises
are given if mobility
limited
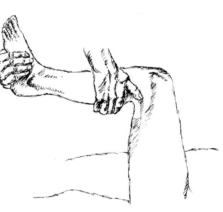

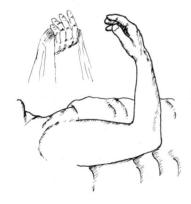

a bedbath is less
tiring for the patient

bed help to prevent sores occurring. Particular attention needs to be paid to the heels. Regular checking of vulnerable areas is vital to prevent redness developing into a sore which is difficult to heal. If there is spasticity it is essential that where the two skin surfaces meet the skin is kept dry and clean. In the final stages a water bed may be necessary.

Nutrition

In the majority of patients this will need to be built up to prevent pressure sores developing and to give greater resistance to infection. Therefore a good nourishing diet will be given with plenty of protein and vitamin C. It will need to be given in small amounts and be easy to handle. Aids may be used to help the patient to hold a glass or cup more securely and if her hands are weak lighter cutlery may make it easier. Assistance will be given with feeding where necessary and a weekly weight chart will give evidence of an increase in weight.

Psychological care

The patient should not be subjected to situations which cause unnecessary stress as these may precipitate or prolong a relapse. The aim is to help her to keep doing those things she enjoys without over exertion. The doctor may order antidepressants or tranquillisers, and if so, the nurse must recognise if the patient is having an adequate amount or needs more. It is essential that all the staff nursing this patient know exactly what she has been told about her condition. Preferably once the diagnosis has been confirmed the doctor will tell her, giving her adequate information. The nurse must have a positive approach, hopeful but not unrealistic. When a remission occurs the patient may think she had been cured, only to find the disease returns. The nurse will need to understand her mood swings and learn to be sensitive to them, helping the patient to recognise her limitations so that she allows others to help her but encouraging her to be as independent as possible and not just adopt the sick role.

Mobility

The aim is to avoid fatigue, and the patient's day will have to be planned carefully to ensure adequate rest periods between periods of activity. Early nights are advisable. During a relapse physiotherapy will mainly consist of passive exercises and maybe light splinting to prevent spasticity. Otherwise the patient will be kept as mobile as possible for as long as possible, without overdoing it. Breathing exercises will be important to prevent chest infection, and weakened muscles, especially those of the arms, need strengthening. If the patient has dizzy spells suitable aids or the assistance of the nurse may promote confidence, and she will need someone to stay with her when she has a bath, although she may find a bed-bath less tiring. A wheelchair is necessary when

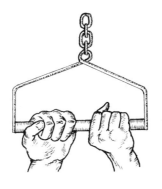

the patient is taught to relieve pressure on the buttocks - a "monkey pole" is useful when confined to bed

check vulnerable areas regularly to avoid the skin breaking - the heels need special care

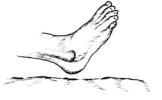

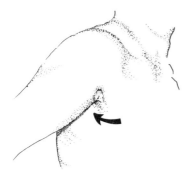

where two skin surfaces meet care is required to keep the patient dry and clean

paraplegia is present or may be used to prevent overtiring. Valium may be ordered by the doctor to control muscle spasm, and the nurse will observe its effectiveness and report, so that adjustments to the dose can be made if necessary.

The patient will be given whatever help she requires with dressing and any adjustments to clothing will be discussed with her and her relatives. Stretchy material, front openings and velcro fastenings will all help her to remain independent for as long as possible. The occupational therapist has an important role in supplying gadgets and showing how clothing may be adjusted, and may also be involved in providing daily living activities.

Continence

If there is any evidence of an urinary infection a midstream specimen of urine will be sent for investigation, fluids will be encouraged, and antibiotics such as Septrin given as prescribed. If the patient is suffering from urgency, she may prefer to be in a bed nearer the toilets and to have a commode at night. Atropine may have been prescribed to reduce bladder irritation and therefore the urgency and frequency. Where there is incontinence it may be possible for the patient to learn how to express the bladder, as catheters are only used if sores are developing and there is no other way to control the incontinence. A change of diet on entering hospital, and reduced activity, may be sufficient to cause constipation even if the patient was not constipated before. Plenty of fruit, vegetables and if necessary the addition of bran will help, as will increased amounts of fluid. It may be necessary to discuss the routine and make alterations in it. Using a bedpan may be inhibitory and it may therefore be preferable for the patient to be wheeled out to the toilet or to have a commode. She may know which aperients are most effective for her and these can then be prescribed by the doctor. Eventually it may be necessary to use suppositories or disposable enemas on a planned basis.

Special senses

Blurring of the vision or double vision will interfere with many activities the patient may wish to do. The nurse will therefore discuss with her and her relatives possible activities she might find interesting. If complete blindness occurs this can be very frightening for the patient, and although it is of a temporary nature will incapacitate her further. When nursing a blind patient care must be taken to explain everything one is doing. As the nurse approaches her she will make the patient aware of this by talking to her. If she is giving her a meal she will ensure that it is something she can handle, explain what it is, and where it is on the plate. Positioning the locker and the things on it will make it easier for the patient to find what she wants without asking. When walking her to the toilet or day room it is better if the patient puts her arm through that of the nurse than the other way round.

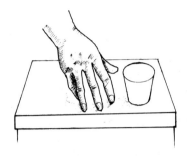

position the locker to
give easy access for
the blind patient

urinary infections require
laboratory examination to
identify the causative organism.
encourage fluids
give prescribed antibiotic

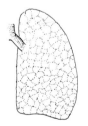

observe patient carefully
for signs of chest infection.
report observations.

Observations

The nurse must be alert to any signs of chest infection and report them immediately. If infection develops the appropriate prescribed antibiotic will be administered by the nurse. Injections may be avoided if she is very thin. She will be nursed as any other pyrexial patient.

Social factors

The hospital social worker will be contacted at an early stage in the patient's admission. Her ability to continue working will be assessed as she may be able to continue in the same job but for less hours once she is discharged. On the other hand if she is in a strenuous occupation it might be advisable for her to give up. Having her own transport will enable her to remain in contact with outside activities for as long as possible, and she may qualify for a mobility allowance. The financial situation will be assessed and whether there is any possibility of a disability allowance or an attendance allowance. If she has young children she may need some assistance with them, which the family itself may be able to provide, otherwise it may be necessary for them to attend a day nursery or nursery school. If she is discharged from hospital on injections of ACTH the district nurse will visit to give these, and if she is paralysed will also bath her and check her pressure areas.

Adaptations to the home such as wider doorways, ramps, and handrails can be carried out by the local authority and enable her to remain at home in a wheel-chair. Relationships within the family need to be assessed, and also the ability of the family to manage without detriment to the patient or themselves, given the necessary help such as a home help or the facilities of a laundry service and supplies of incontinent pads where required. It should always be possible for the patient to be readmitted to hospital if the situation warrants it.

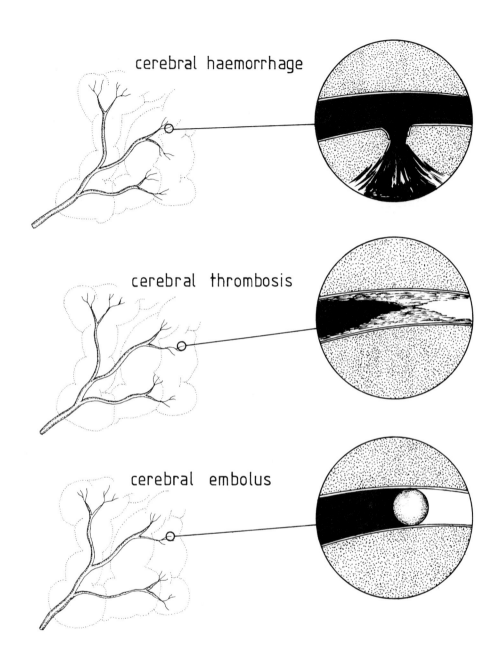

37 Cerebrovascular accident

PATHOLOGY

From each of the three main cerebral arteries there are branches to
the deeper substance of the brain. If one of these ruptures or
becomes blocked, oxygen cannot reach the part of the brain supplied by it which will therefore die or become infarcted. If the blood
vessel supplying the internal capsule is affected then there will be a
profound hemiplegia on the opposite side of the body to the lesion.
Because the neurones from the brain to the spinal cord are affected,
this is an upper motor neurone lesion, and although in the first few
weeks there will be a flaccid paralysis on the affected side, once
spinal shock has worn off there will be a spastic paralysis with exaggerated reflexes. This is because the control of the reflexes by the
brain has been lost.

Cerebral haemorrhage
The walls of the arteries in the brain may be weak due to atheroma
or an aneurysm and the pressure within them increased due to
hypertension. Any further rise in pressure, for example due to
bouts of severe coughing or emotional crises may be sufficient to
rupture the blood vessel and cause a cerebral haemorrhage. If not
fatal, the clot may fibrose over, but there is always danger of it rup-
turing, especially in the early days. A cerebral haemorrhage results
in a deeply unconscious patient. The death rate is high and the recovery rate poor as there is usually a profound paralysis.

Cerebral thrombosis
Plaques of atheroma gradually build up on the arteries throughout
the body and the site of the first incident will depend on where the
deposits are greatest. The patient could develop ischaemic heart
disease, intermittent claudication, or cerebral ischaemia or thrombosis. The narrowed roughened surface of the artery allows the
build up of a thrombus which will eventually block the vessel.
Before a thrombus actually forms, there may be a period when the
patient has episodes of mental confusion due to a diminished blood
supply to the brain. Once the thrombus has formed there will be
death of the tissue supplied. The recovery of the patient will
depend on the extent of the brain tissue involved.

Cerebral embolus
In subacute bacterial endocarditis, auricular fibrillation, or a
mural thrombosis following a myocardial infaction, a clot or
embolus may be thrown off which will travel in the general circulation until it reaches a blood vessel small enough to block its progress. It may of course go to many other organs of the body but

associated with obesity

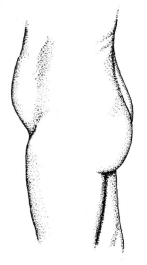

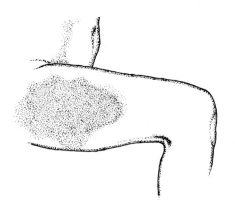

bruising may be present

consciousness will   vary

70 blood pressure falls

frequently travels to the brain so causing a blockage in its blood supply. These patients will obviously have a history of one of the conditions mentioned, and may have a history of embolic episodes. As with a haemorrhage it occurs suddenly, but tends to be of short duration and the recovery from a particular incident is good.

NURSING ASSESSMENT

This patient may be admitted deeply unconscious, and therefore the nurse will have to gain her information from the relatives and her own observations. Even if the patient is conscious his speech may be affected so interfering with communication.

General appearance
One would expect the patient to be over fifty; a younger patient might suggest an embolus. Both obesity and a florid complexion may be present.

Condition of the skin
There may be bruising or abrasions from falling, but one would not expect pressures sores unless the patient had been at home for some time.

Mental state
The patient may be in any of the stages of unconsciousness described under that heading, or fully conscious. In the latter case he may be emotionally unstable, easily dissolving into tears, as a result of frustration or fear. The relatives, if present when the attack occurred, may be able to say whether there were any warning signs such as a headache, slurred speech, or periods of confusion. The patient may have complained of dizziness or faint-ness. It is important to find out what the patient was like before the attack.

Mobility
In the initial stages it is expected that the reflexes will be absent but after the first few weeks they will become exaggerated. The nurse will note the ability of the patient to move his limbs and react to sen-sation.

Excretion
The bladder should be palpated to see if it is full, and an assessment made as to whether there is incontinence or retention with over-flow. Diabetes predisposes to a cerebrovascular accident, and therefore the urine should be checked for sugar. Incontinence of faeces, constipation, or spurious diarrhoea may be present.

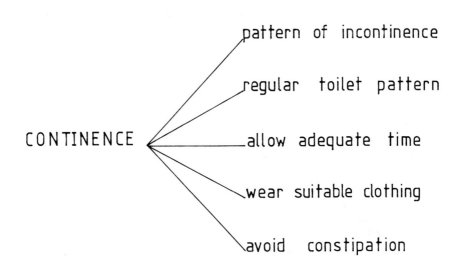

CONTINENCE
- pattern of incontinence
- regular toilet pattern
- allow adequate time
- wear suitable clothing
- avoid constipation

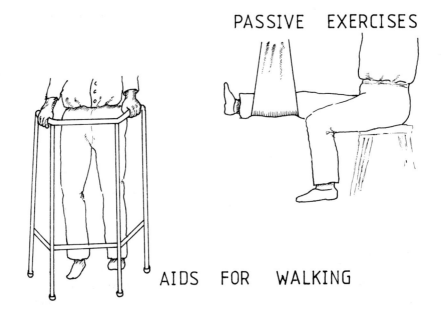

PASSIVE EXERCISES

AIDS FOR WALKING

Special senses
If the patient is conscious he may have difficulty in seeing due to **hemianopia,** loss of half the vision in each eye, corresponding to the side affected by the paralysis. **Nystagmus,** rapid movements of the eye, may be present. In the conscious patient it will be necessary to assess the patient's speech and his understanding. Does he know what he wants but is unable to say it, or does he give objects the wrong name.

Observations
The blood pressure will probably be low even if the patient suffered from hypertension prior to the attack. If there is damage in the region of the hypothalamus there will be hyperpyrexia. Noisy breathing indicates airway obstruction. Shallow breathing or **Cheyne–Stokes respiration** may also be noted.

NURSING CARE PLAN

In the initial period the patient with a cerebrovascular accident may be unconscious. If this is so then the relevant care will be given, as is described in Chapter 34. The aim at that time is not to allow any complication to occur which will hinder progress at a later stage. As the patient regains conciousness the nursing care plan will be evaluated and readjusted accordingly. The aim in the second stage will be to restore as much of the original function as is possible.

Care of the skin
The patient will be encouraged to become as independent as possible and may find it preferable to sit down under a shower than to be helped in and out of a bath even with rails and special seats. Many patients feel insecure in a hoist. He will need assistance with cutting toe nails and finger nails. Short hair is obviously easier to manage than long if one hand is out of action. Care of the pressure areas will remain important while there is any restriction on mobility and care must be taken to protect the paralysed limbs from injury due to contact with hot surfaces or being in an abnormal position.

Nutrition
As soon as the patient is able he should be encouraged to feed himself. However care will need to be taken to monitor that he is having an adequate diet, as he may give up before he has had sufficient. It is easier for him to eat if he is sitting out at a table well supported. Initially it is better for him to remain by his bed so that if he does make a mess others are not watching. Adequate protection is essential although bibs may be thought to be demoralising. Special plates with an outer rim and cutlery with large handles can be pro-

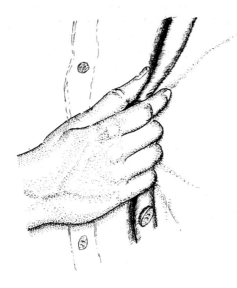

clothing can be adapted
to make dressing
easier for the patient

A PLANNED PROGRAMME WILL HELP
THE PATIENT REGAIN MANUAL SKILLS

special aids are
available to
assist the
patient when
dressing; allow the patient plenty of time to
put on his clothes

vided, and these can be put on a non slip plastic mat. There are a variety of non-spill cups which the patient might find useful. The best way of using the equipment should be explained to the patient, and assistance given as necessary. The diet needs to be kept interesting, and not just mince and fish, but it should suitable and where necessary cut up. It is also necessary to to keep a careful check on the amount of fluid taken in as it may be too much effort for the patient to drink sufficient. With paralysis on one side, food accumulates in that cheek, and it is therefore essential to clean the mouth after a meal.

Psychological care

These patients are easily depressed or over-excited and may also feel that the responsibility for their recovery rests with the medical and nursing staff and not with themselves. Although antidepressants may be used to control the depression, it is the nurses and relatives who can give most support. Tolerance of stress and frustration is limited, and therefore the nurse needs to be able to assess the right moment to step in and help. Short term, easily attainable goals need to be set, and the relatives kept in the picture so that they can reinforce the treatment.

Mobility

As soon as the patient is fit to get up he will be mobilised. When standing he should be encouraged to straighten up and look ahead. When walking the affected foot has a tendency to drag on the ground and therefore calipers with a strong spring to lift the foot may be necessary. He must be well supported when sitting, aiming to keep as good a posture as possible, with pillows placed strategically. Care will need to be taken when lifting him as incorrect lifting may do damage to joints which will prolong his recovery. Physiotherapy, progressing through passive to active exercises will be started early. When the patient is able to go down to the department he will receive his treatment there. Initially this will consist of passive exercises in supporting slings, and gradually the patient will progress to exercises in walking and games involving balance and co-ordination, so that some of his therapy will be on an individual basis and some within groups. He may progress from using a tripod as an aid to walking to a walking stick, from walking on a flat surface to walking on a rough uneven surface, and eventually manage slopes and stairs including a bus step. All the time the physiotherapist is making the best use of muscles which are still functional, and trying to restore as much function to the others as possible.

Dressing

The occupational therapist in conjunction with the nurse will assess what the patient can do and then will plan the succeeding programme the patient is to follow. This is one activity the relatives

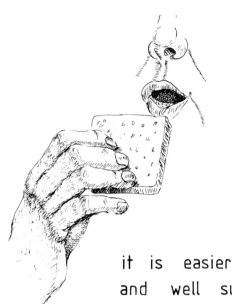

patients should be
encouraged to feed
themselves

it is easier if seated at a table
and well supported in a chair

use adequate protection of the
patient - and avoid embarrassment
by allowing the patient privacy

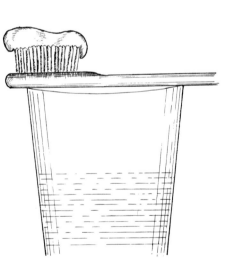

keep the mouth
and teeth clean
after each meal

might like to assist in. Undressing is easier to do than dressing, so it is better to start with this to help the patient gain confidence. The clothing may have to be adapted to make it easier for him to dress. Stretchy material is better than woven, front openings are easier to manage particularly on garments like brassieres, and velcro fastenings are not as difficult as hooks and eyes. Elastic shoe laces and buttons sewn on with elastic overcome impossible tasks. There are numerous gadgets which can be used by the patient where he cannot manage on his own, such as extra long shoe horns to help put a shoe on and aids to put stockings or tights on.

It is important to allow the patient plenty of time to dress or he will become flustered and therefore less able. The occupational therapist, from her wide experience of such patients, will be able to make suggestions which will make the task easier. The patient needs to be told that when dressing he should put the affected arm into the garment first, whereas when undressing he should take the good arm out first. When putting garments on the lower half it will be easier if he crosses the affected leg over the other knee. A jumper or similar garment can be taken off by catching hold of the back of the collar and pulling the garment over the head. The patient should wear his own clothes which will enhance his sense of well-being. Facilities may need to be made available for laundering, unless the relatives can manage.

Progress will then be made onto daily living activities. A simulated kitchen, bathroom and workshop will be available to the patient once he reaches an adequate standard of mobility. In this unit the occupational therapist will assess what type of assistance and equipment will be of use. If necessary the social worker will make arrangements for alterations to be made in the home.

Continence
The sooner the patient can control bladder and bowel function the better for his morale. A pattern of his incontinence will be made, the patient then being regularly toileted at the appropriate times. Once the patient is walking he should be encouraged to go out to the toilet in plenty of time, as he has not the same control over sphincters. Raised toilets, and handrails, will help to give him confidence. Clothing will need to be easily handled, but this is not a reason for leaving off undergarments. The doctor will examine the patient to check for impacted faeces or urinary infection. If either of these is present they will be treated. A mild aperient or suppositories may be used for constipation.

Communication
The speech therapist will work with the patient if speech is affected, discovering his problems and assisting him to overcome them. When talking to such a patient the nurse should ask short direct questions which have only one answer to them.

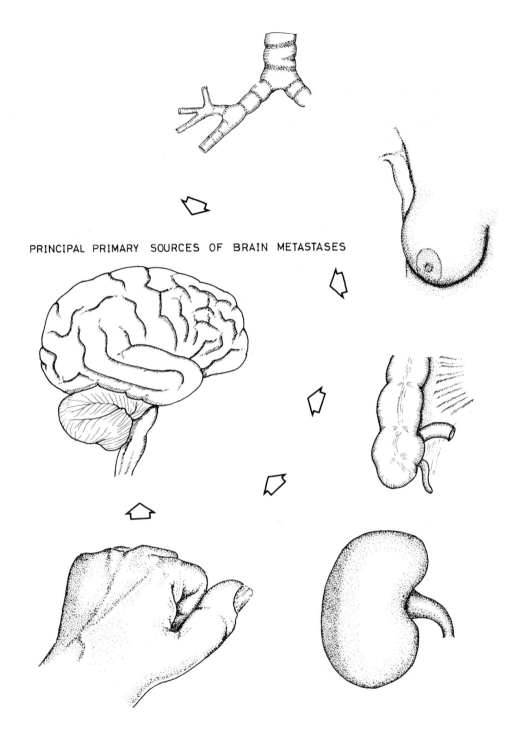

PRINCIPAL PRIMARY SOURCES OF BRAIN METASTASES

38 Brain tumours

PATHOLOGY

Because neurones have a limited ability to regenerate, tumours arising from these cells are very rare. They do occur in the cerebellum in children, and in this case are inoperable, being treated by radiotherapy. They may also arise in the ganglia of the autonomic nervous system and the medulla of the adrenal gland. Those tumours developing in the central nervous system more commonly arise from the glial cells (supporting connective tissue) and are called **gliomas.** They are given their name according to the type of cell affected. They spread locally but do not usually metastasise. However, except for those arising in the meninges, known as **meningiomas,** they cannot be removed completely, if at all, so that eventually considerable brain damage will occur. Although they may grow very slowly it is more common for them to grow rapidly. Some tumours form cysts which can be drained, so relieving some pressure. Radiotherapy is therefore a palliative measure.

The most common neoplasms of the brain are carcinomatous metastases from a primary growth in other parts of the body such as the bronchus, breast, gastrointestinal tract, kidneys or skin. Most of these occur in the cerebrum although some occur in the cerebellum and the brain stem.

Some tumours because of their position press on vital structures such as the cranial nerves and therefore produce specific signs. Thus an **acoustic neuroma** will press on the eighth cranial nerve so causing deafness. It may also press on seventh and fifth cranial nerves causing facial paralysis and numbness, and on the cerebellum resulting in ataxia, disorders of speech and nystagmus. Tumours of the pituitary gland may press on the nearby optic nerve causing a bitemporal hemianopia and eventually blindness. Pituitary tumours can also cause endocrine dysfunction, leading to acromegaly or Cushing's syndrome.

Investigations
Skull X-rays, electroencephalogram, ventriculogram, radioisotope brain scan, computerised axial tomography (CAT scan).

Treatment
Magnesium sulphate, intravenous mannitol, and steroids such as dexamethasone may be given to obtain a rapid reduction of intracranial pressure. Surgery and radiotherapy are the main lines of treatment.

drooping of the
face and eyelid

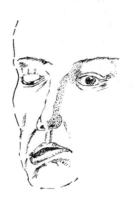

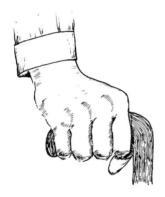

unsteady gait
(ataxia)

transient blurring
of vision
(papilloedema)

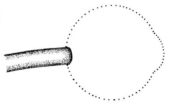

A brain tumour may develop so insidiously that early signs and symptoms are missed. Abnormalities may be overlooked particularly when the individual is not personally known. Therefore the relatives are an important source of information.

General appearance
The general condition of the patient may indicate that he has not been eating adequately, and on questioning it may be found that he has a poor appetite, or suffers from attacks of vomiting. There may be drooping of the face and eyelid on one side, indicating paralysis.

Condition of the skin
If there is sensory impairment of the skin then there may be sores and abrasions of which he is unaware.

Mental state
A tumour in the region of the cerebrum will lead to a deterioration of mental ability. There may be some difficulty in grasping what is said, not because of poor hearing but due to a lack of understanding and loss of memory. Personality changes will also occur causing argumentative and irrational behaviour. There may also be a deterioration in social behaviour. Gradually as the tumour enlarges the patient will complain of increasing headaches which are worse lying down. He will become progressively more drowsy until comatose.

Mobility
Damage to the motor pathways from the brain will lead to hemiparesis and hemiplegia, whereas tumours in the region of the cerebellum cause an unsteady gait (ataxia).

Excretion
Incontinence may be present.

Special senses
If the optic nerves are involved, hemianopia, double vision, or even loss of vision, may be complained of. On examination the pupils may be seen to be dilated and have a sluggish reaction to light. They may also appear to move rapidly (nystagmus). On examination with the ophthalmascope the doctor will see papilloedema which may cause episodes of transient blurring of vision.

Hearing will be affected if the tumour is in the region of the auditory nerve. It is particularly important to notice any difficulties the patient has in talking and answering questions. He may have difficulty in finding the right words, in understanding or physically saying what he wants. His speech may be incoherent or slurred.

125

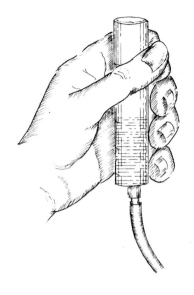

when <u>conscious</u> :-
encourage to eat.
when <u>unconscious</u> :-
  <u>1</u>. naso-gastric tube
    feeding.
  <u>2</u>. intravenous feeding.

increase pressure
area care when
patient is confined
to bed.

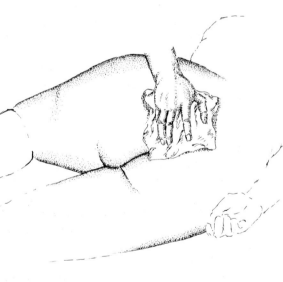

Observations

As intracranial pressure rises so will the blood pressure, the pulse slowing. Pressure near the medulla oblongata will affect the heart and respiratory rates.

NURSING CARE PLAN

As the patient's condition progresses there will need to be continual adaptation of the nursing care.

Care of the skin

If the patient is having deep X-ray treatment to the brain his head may be shaved, and the skin will need particular care to prevent its breakdown. As the patient becomes confined to bed, pressure area care becomes increasingly important.

Nutrition

If the patient is suffering from nausea and vomiting an anti-emetic will be prescribed by the doctor, and he will be encouraged to eat those foods which he can tolerate more easily. As he becomes unconscious a nasogastric tube and intravenous therapy will be required. Fluids are usually restricted to one or one and a half litres in 24 hours.

Psychological care

Analgesics will be prescribed by the doctor for headaches. These should be adequate but not so much as to make the patient drowsy. If the patient is restless and irritable, sedatives will also have been prescribed, and antidepressives if required. Maintaining the patient at home for as long as possible will help to minimise depression, but the relatives will need adequate support and advice. When diminishing consciousness is combined with restlessness cotsides will be necessary.

Mobility

The aim is to keep the patient as mobile as possible for as long as possible. Where there is paralysis and therefore impaired mobility, aids and appliances will be used. Because this patient frequently becomes irritated and frustrated it may difficult for him to accept his limitations and adapt his life accordingly.

Continence

Incontinence may arise due to impaired mobility or lack of awareness, or because the nerve pathways have been damaged. The cause must be found and the method of management will vary accordingly. Regular toileting may be sufficient, but if nerve pathways are damaged catheterisation may be necessary. A pituitary tumour may cause excessive loss of urine and therefore a fluid chart

THE SPECIAL SENSES

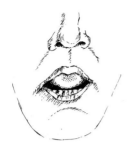

speech therapy may be
given if patient has
difficulty in expressing himself

irrigation may be needed if
patient has difficulty in
closing his eyelids

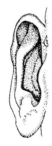

it is important to communicate
if the patient becomes deaf

urinary output
must be measured
and recorded

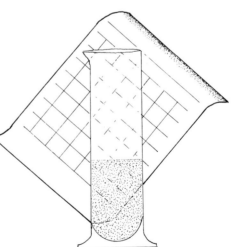

will be necessary. If the patient is on steroids the urine will be tested for sugar. A careful watch will have to kept for constipation particularly if the patient is on analgesics with this side effect.

Special senses
If there is deteriorating vision the patient may not be able to read or even watch television, and may therefore appreciate someone reading to him. If there is any difficulty in closing the eyes, regular irrigation will be necessary. Any deafness will add to the feeling of isolation, and therefore, however difficult it is to communicate with the patient, an effort should be made to include him in the conversation. This should be explained to the relatives as well. Speech therapy will be necessary if the patient has any difficulty in expressing himself, and the therapist will also be able to give both the nurses and relatives advice on how they may best help the patient.

Observations
If the patient is on steroids infection may be masked, and he is particularly prone to it if he is receiving radiotherapy. Therefore the patient should be observed carefully for any indication of infection. Not only should the temperature be taken but difficulty in breathing and chesty sounds also noted. Neurological observations will be carried out, their frequency depending on the state of the patient. Any changes in the mental state of the patient will be recorded, as will changes in personality. The relatives can be very helpful in this as they will be aware at an early stage of these changes.

extradural
haemorrhage

intracranial
haemorrhage

subdural
haemorrhage

concussion

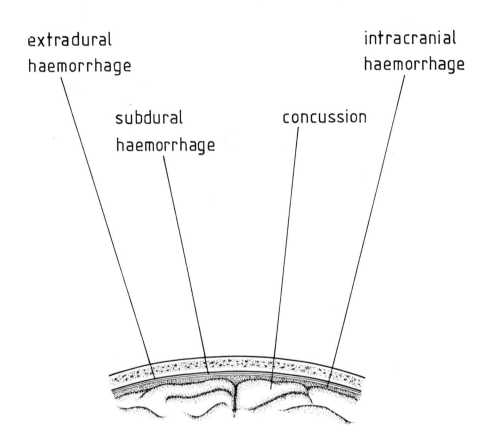

HEAD   INJURY

39 Head injury

PATHOLOGY

After trauma to the head the effects may be immediate as in concussion or extradural haemorrhage; Symptoms may arise a few days later as in meningitis, subdural haemorrhage or chest complications; or sometimes the effects occur some years later as with epileptic fits due to scarring of the brain.

Extradural haemorrhage

This condition is most likely to occur in the younger patient, and is bleeding between the skull and the dura due to a ruptured **middle meningeal artery** which is just inside the skull. It can extend quickly and if not treated will cause death. Casualties may or may not lose consciousness initially, and if they do, they regain it quickly. After an hour, or at the most two, the patient complains of an increasingly severe headache, becoming progressively more drowsy. He may develop a hemiplegia. The pupil on the damaged side becomes larger, the blood pressure rises, and the pulse slows. If not treated both pupils dilate and the patient dies. If the clot is removed early enough by suction through burr holes the patient will recover with no ill effects.

Subdural haemorrhage

In order for a young person to suffer from this type of haemorrhage the blow would probably have to be sufficient to fracture the skull. However in the elderly the brain has become smaller in relation to the skull and therefore there is more movement allowing vessels to be pulled and ruptured, causing a haemorrhage between the arachnoid and duramater. A blow on one side of the head will cause the brain to hit the other side of the skull and rebound (**contrecoup injury**). Therefore the damage may be on the opposite side to the blow. The clinical picture is similar to that in an extradural haemorrhage but takes days or weeks to develop. The patient will complain of a headache of increasing severity, become increasingly drowsy, and may also have fits due to the cerebral irritation. Again the treatment is to evacuate the clot.

Concussion

If the impact at the time of injury is considerable, the person will become unconscious for a variable amount of time. As he recovers he may be confused, restless, irritable and possibly violent. The effects in some people may continue for some time after the initial incident, the person complaining of headaches, dizziness or difficulty in concentration, but eventually there is full recovery.

fractures   to   base   of   the
skull

raised   intracranial   pressure
causing   coning

[damaging   reticular   formation &   vital centres]

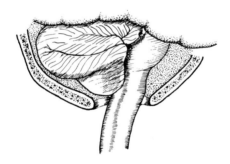

Brain   Stem   Damage

Intracranial haemorrhage

This may occur if there is a depressed fracture of the skull or a penetrating wound. The patient may be deeply unconscious but so long as his general condition is maintained, he may recover even after weeks. However unless he is very young there will probably be some degree of physical or mental handicap. If he is over 25 recovery is unlikely.

Damage to the brain stem

This occurs due to fractures at the base of the skull and frequently causes profound coma and death. This is because the **reticular formation** responsible for maintaining alertness is in the brain stem. Damage to the **vital centres** in the medulla oblongata will cause instant death. Another important cause of damage to the brain stem is **coning.** This occurs when raised intracranial pressure forces the cerebrum down through the opening in the cranial cavity, so pressing on the brain stem. Again the reticular formation and the vital centres will become damaged, leading to coma and death.

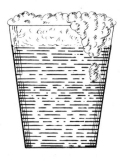

look for evidence of
drink or drugs

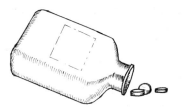

observe   for   bruising
measure   the girth at
regular   intervals

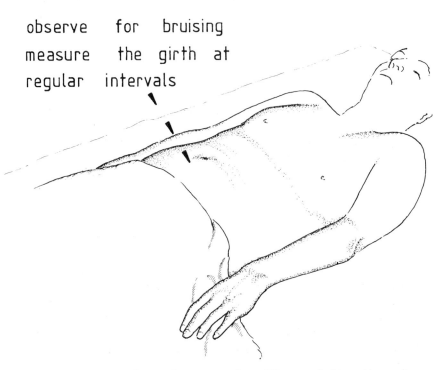

listen for bowel sounds [? paralytic ileus]

Information about the head injury patient will almost certainly need to be gained from observers, and usually this will be the ambulance driver. It is essential to find out from him the patient's level of consciousness immediately after the accident and if there has been any change in this.

General appearance

The patient may be a young healthy adult, or an elderly individual, the former having a better chance of recovery and presenting fewer physical and social problems. There may be evidence of drinking alcohol or drug taking. The whole body should be examined carefully for evidence of further injury. The limbs will be noted for their position, any abnormality indicating a fracture, and any bruising over the abdomen especially in the region of the liver will indicate abdominal bleeding. The girth will have to be measured at regular intervals to check for any increase, and bowel sounds will also be listened for as paralytic ileus may occur. Any skin abrasions or lacerations will be noted, particularly if present on the scalp as these may indicate a compound fracture. Evidence of paralysis when the patient tries to move will also be noted.

Mental state

The patient will be assessed for level of consciousness, estimated by response to painful stimuli or the spoken command. Account will be taken of what his condition was like before admission. If the patient is not unconscious then the nurse will observe his behaviour, noting whether he is rational, restless or irritable. The patient may develop twitching due to hyperventilation, or even have actual epileptiform fits. The nurse must observe these carefully as described in Chapter 40 on epilepsy.

Excretion

The patient should be checked to see if there is any incontinence. If the bladder is full and there is no incontinence this suggests damage to the spinal cord. Excessive output may occur due to damage to the pituitary causing diabetes inspidus, or conversely a reduced amount of urine may indicate acute renal failure. If there is damage to the urinary tract haematuria may be present. The urine will be tested for sugar in particular, as the accident could have been the result of disturbance in consciousness due to hypoglycaemia.

rising pulse

falling blood
pressure

SHOCK

slow bounding
pulse

rising blood
pressure

RISING INTRA-
CRANIAL PRESSURE

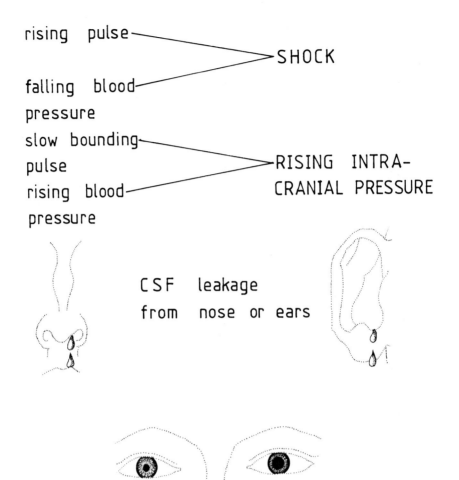

CSF leakage
from nose or ears

size and equality of the pupils,
and their response to light

OBSERVATIONS IN HEAD INJURY

Observations

The breathing will be assessed to see whether it is noisy, indicating a partial obstruction which may occur due to a denture, the tongue or secretions. The depth of respirations is also important, as it may be too shallow to be adequate, or there may be hyperventilation leading to loss of carbon dioxide. If the pulse is rising and the blood pressure falling it suggests that shock is developing due to another injury. If however the pulse becomes slow and bounding and the blood pressure rises this indicates rising intracranial pressure. In both cases medical atention is needed. A baseline must be established on admission in order to compare the patient's progress. The temperature may be raised if the damage is in the region of the hypothalamus. Neurological observations will be carried out. In a fracture of base of skull there may be leakage of cerebrospinal fluid from the nose or ear. As a result of this communication between the meninges and the outside, meningitis is likely to develop later. If there is any vomiting, the amount will be noted, and whether it is effortless or associated with much retching. Any blood in the vomitus will suggest internal bleeding, and if there is any suspicion of drug taking then a specimen will be sent to the laboratory.

Social factors

The police will have checked to see if there is any information regarding the patient's relatives and will have informed them, but the nurse is responsible for checking that this has been done. Any identity bracelet, Medic Alert bracelet, or card indicating that the patient is on drugs such as anticoagulants or steroids, or has a condition such as diabetes or epilepsy, should have been looked for.

MAINTAIN A CLEAR AIRWAY

may require :-

endotracheal tube
tracheostomy

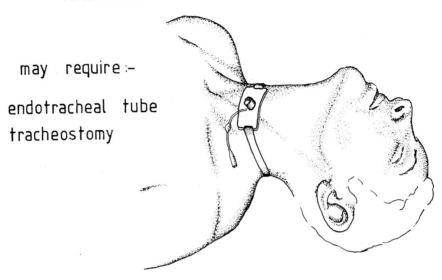

MAINTAIN FLUID BALANCE

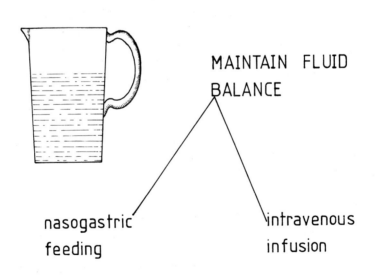

nasogastric
feeding

intravenous
infusion

The patient is frequently unconscious, and therefore the nurse will be relying on observations to note any changes. Initially the care will be that of the unconscious patient as described earlier in the book, but with particular emphasis on certain aspects which will be discussed here.

Maintenance of the airway

If respiration is inadequate due to very shallow breathing the doctor will need to be informed as it may be necessary to pass an endotracheal tube, or to perform a tracheostomy if ventilation is required for more than 24 hours. Suction is important to remove secretions obstructing the airway. Hyperventilation will lead to a loss of carbon dioxide resulting in alkalosis and tetany. Therefore if it occurs the doctor will order a drug such as morphia to depress the respiratory centre. Chest infection frequently occurs in the patient with a head injury in which case antibiotics may be ordered.

Observations

The pulse may be rapid at first due to shock, and as the patient recovers fall to normal limits. If it remains fast and weak this suggests bleeding in some other part of the body. If it continues to fall below normal it is an indication of increasing intracranial pressure. Likewise a low blood pressure indicates shock initially, and if it persists, haemorrhage. A rising blood pressure occurs with increased intracranial pressure. These must therefore be assessed at regular intervals, possibly at quarter hourly intervals at first, but less frequently as the patient progresses. If shock is present the foot of the bed should be raised. If it is suspected that haemorrhage is present, the doctor will examine the patient to find out exactly where it is and whether surgical intervention is necessary. Pyrexia, particularly when there is damage in the region of the hypothalamus, will require measures to reduce it such as tepid sponging or a fan. Antipyretic drugs such as aspirin may also be ordered. Neurological observations will be continued and observation for fits which may be controlled by diazepam.

Nutrition

An adequate intake of fluid is vital to the head injury patient. Any sign of metabolic disturbance, pyrexia or hyperventilation will mean that the patient is losing more fluid from the body and this must be replaced. It may be necessary to give as much as two to three litres in 24 hours. This will probably be given via a nasogastric tube unless the patient is vomiting. A proportion of the fluids may be given intravenously, particularly if there is to be replacement of electrolytes or the administration of intravenous drugs. Antiemetic drugs such as Fentazin may be necessary to control vomiting. Intravenous mannitol can be given to reduce a

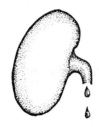

observe and record
urinary output

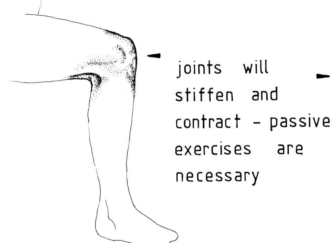

joints will
stiffen and
contract - passive
exercises are
necessary

NEUROLOGICAL OBSERVATIONS ARE
MAINTAINED

raised intracranial pressure, but if it is, fluid will have to be monitored carefully. Calorie intake must be adequate, bearing in mind that a raised temperature and increased metabolic rate will use up more calories. A well-balanced diet containing 2250 kilocalories a day can be adjusted according to the patient's specific requirements. Distilled water is sometimes used instead of tap water to keep the level of calcium low because of the tendency for renal stones to form. For the same reason liquidised foods are preferred to manufactured foods as these are often high in calcium.

Mobility
Unless passive exercises are carried out by the physiotherapist and nurses the joints will become stiff and contract, so making mobilisation at a later date more difficult.

Continence
Renal stones may form in the urinary tract so leading to urinary infection, therefore adequate fluids must be given. Evidence of infection must be recognised early or pyelonephritis and damage to the kidney will occur. Observation of the renal output may also reveal a reduced volume of urine following severe shock, indicating that the patient has gone into renal failure, and may require urgent dialysis.

Relatives
When the relatives arrive they will probably be in a distraught state, and may require to be calmed down and given careful explanations before they see the patient. Any equipment around the patient is likely to worry them, and so full explanations of why it is necessary and that these are routine measures may help to reassure them. If the patient has unsightly lacerations, bruising or oedema they will need to be told that this is not as bad as it appears and will subside. False hopes must not be raised, but on the other hand one should not be too pessimistic. If the patient is considered to be dangerously ill, then the close relatives may wish to remain at the hospital, and suitable arrangements will have to be made.

Evaluation
As the patient's condition progresses so his nursing care plan will need to be adjusted. Recovery of consciousness may bring with its restlessness, confusion or even violence. Restriction should be kept to a minimum. Cot sides may be necessary although if the patient persists in climbing over these he may be better nursed on a mattress on the floor temporarily. At this time he must be watched carefully, or he may do further damage to himself.

EPILEPSY

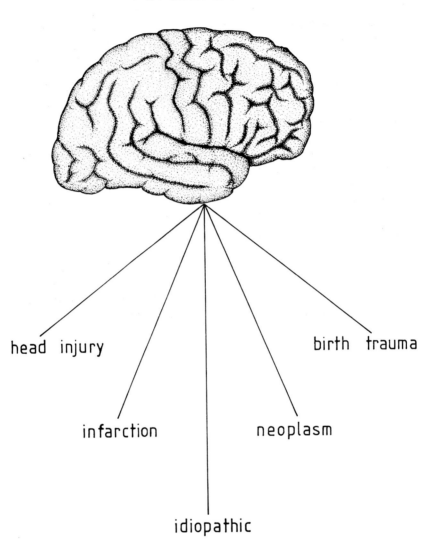

head injury   birth trauma

    infarction   neoplasm

              idiopathic

40 Epilepsy

PATHOLOGY

Epilepsy is the name given to the condition in which an individual has recurring fits arising from a sudden abnormal activity of the brain. It is thought that this may be due to biochemical changes. Epilepsy is not a disease in the true sense, because it can only be said to be present when the individual is actually having fits.

Epileptiform fits may occur following a head injury in an adult or after a difficult birth in an infant, where scar tissue has formed in the brain. For the same reason a brain infarction arising from a blocked or damaged blood vessel may also cause fits. Another cause may be pressure on the brain from any type of tumour, but in the majority of people suffering from epilepsy there appears to be no apparent cause and it is therefore called **idiopathic epilepsy.** There often appears to be a family history of the condition. It is considered that nerve cells will become disorganised under certain stimuli and that some people have a lower threshold than others, the level of the threshold being inherited. Alcohol appears to increase the susceptibility of the cells. Precipitating factors may be hypoglycaemia, pregnancy, strong emotional states such as fear, anger or shock, flashing lights, high fever (especially in children), lack of oxygen, lack of sleep and overhydration. An electroencephalogram (EEG) is normal in the majority of cases, although there is a characteristic pattern when fits occur.

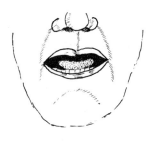

may experience a taste
or smell - an AURA

followed by loss of
consciousness, muscle
rigidity, clenched jaws
and cyanosis
the TONIC stage.

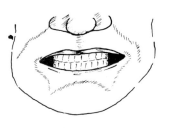

Followed by involuntary jerking movements
the CLONIC stage

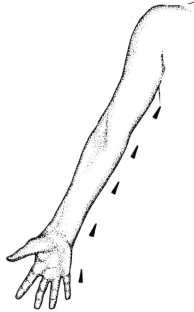

in Jacksonian epilepsy
the jerking movement
follows a definite
pattern

Grand mal fits

The patient may have some kind of warning, either just a sense that something is going to happen, or a change of mood which is called a **prodrome,** or he may experience a taste, smell, or visual disturbance, an **aura.** But he may have no warning at all.

He then loses consciousness becoming completely rigid, with muscles contracted and jaws clenched. Air being forced out of the lungs through the vocal cords may cause a cry. There will be cyanosis. This is the **tonic** stage.

Following this there are involuntary jerking movements during which the patient may bite his tongue. It is at this stage that the patient may be incontinent of urine or even faeces, due to contraction of the abdominal muscles. This is called the **clonic** stage.

A deep sleep follows, which may be only brief but could last as long as two hours. Following the fit the patient is not aware of what has happened and will probably not know where he is. He may complain of a headache and may remain sleepy or confused. Occasionally there is a period of automatism in which the patient is unaware of what he is doing.

Petit mal attacks

This condition mainly affects children between the ages of five and twelve years and consists of brief lapses of consciousness when the child does not appear to be attending. They may be so brief they pass unnoticed. During the attack the child will stop what he is doing and may drop anything he is holding. If he is talking there will be a pause and he will have a vacant stare with fluttering of the eyelids.

Jacksonian fits

The involuntary movements follow a definite pattern, starting in the fingers and travelling up the arm to the shoulder.

Focal Epilepsy

This is due to a localised lesion of the brain which causes it to produce a particular pattern, as with **temporal lobe epilepsy** where the aura may be one of taste or smell.

Status epilepticus

When a series of epileptic fits follows one after another without the patient regaining consciousness this is called status epilepticus. The temperature rises and the patient may die due to hyperpyrexia or exhaustion.

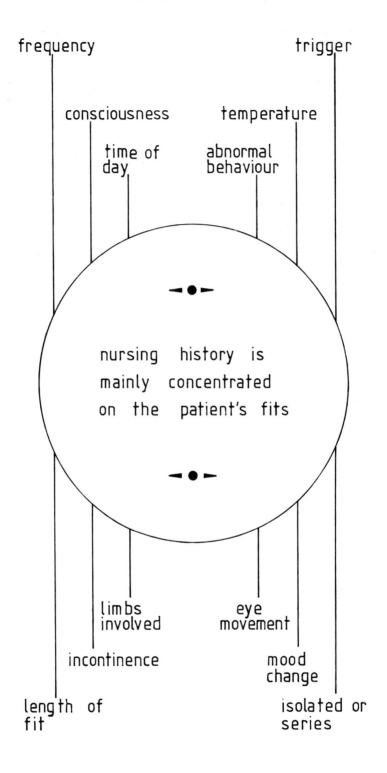

frequency

trigger

consciousness

temperature

time of
day

abnormal
behaviour

nursing   history   is
mainly   concentrated
on   the   patient's   fits

limbs
involved

eye
movement

incontinence

mood
change

length   of
fit

isolated or
series

Because epilepsy is not a disease causing permanent changes the nursing history will probably not show any significant problems. There may be evidence of trauma to the body due to falls from previous fits. This section will therefore concentrate on an assessment of the fits. If an individual suffers from fits the following information will be needed, some of which may best be obtained from a relative who has observed the fits.

How often do the fits occur and over what period of time?
Is there anything that appears to trigger them off?
Is consciousness lost?
Is the temperature raised?
Do the fits occur at a certain time in the day, or do they appear to occur when meals are missed or late?
Is there any abnormal behaviour either before or after the fit?
Do the fits start on one side or with a particular limb?
Is there any mood change or aura prior to the fit?
Do the eyes move in a particular direction?
Is there any incontinence?
How long do the fits last?
Are they isolated attacks or a series of fits at one time?

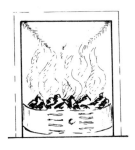

remove potential danger
from patient's environment,
unguarded fires or sharp
edges

protect the head
from injury

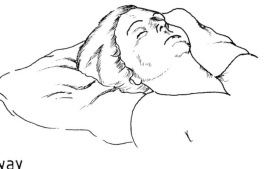

support the angle
of the jaw and
maintain the airway

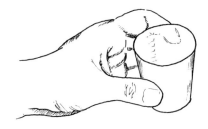

ensure that drugs
are given at the
prescribed times

If a patient has a fit the following care needs to be taken.

Remove any potential danger, such as sharp edges, away from the patient.

If necessary remove the patient from danger area, for example a fire.

Do not restrain.

Maintain the airway, usually by supporting the angle of the jaw until involuntary movements cease and the patient can be placed in the semiprone position.

Place something under the head to protect it from knocks.

If anything is placed in the mouth, this should be soft to prevent damage to the teeth, and would not be put in the mouth during the tonic stage.

After the fit the patient should be told that he has had a fit, where he is and that there is someone there to care for him.

Leave him to sit or lie quietly but keep under observation until confident that he is completely aware of what he is doing.

Any incontinence must be dealt with.

Medication

Grand mal

Phenobarbitone (Luminal) 100–300 mg daily

Primidone (Mysoline) 250–2000 mg daily

Phenytoin sodium (Epanutin, Dilantin) 300–600 mg daily

Phenobarbitone and primidone will cause sleepiness if given in high doses, the aim is therefore to bring the fits under control without diminishing alertness. Phenytoin causes hyperplasia of the gums and may therefore interfere with the dental development of children.

Petit mal

Troxidone (Tridione) 600–1200 mg daily

This may affect the eyes, causing day blindness, or the kidneys, causing nephrotic syndrome, and may precipitate blood disorders.

Status epilepticus

Diazepam IV slowly (up to 10 mg/min) 0·25–0·75 mg per kilogram body weight OR one of the following:

Sodium phenytoin IM or IV.   Sodium phenobarbitone IM

Paraldehyde IM or IV   Thiopentone IV

Lignocaine IV

A Medic Alert bracelet should be worn, and a supply of tablets always carried.

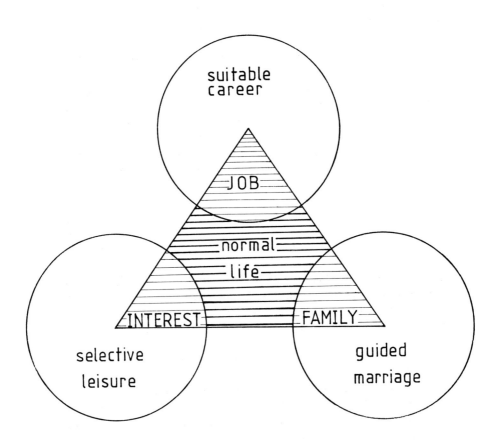

Advice

The more normal and interesting a life the individual leads the less fits he is likely to have. There must be a sensible balance between the risks and restrictions. Certain risks are unjustifiable, but over-protection can be just as damaging to a developing personality. The decision to tell other people will depend on whether they may have to deal with a fit, although there should not be a conspiracy of silence about the condition, and it should not be kept from the child. Epileptics who only have fits at night, or are completely controlled by drugs may feel that it is unnecessary to inform their employers. Advice should be given on how to deal with the fits.

Vocational: The disablement resettlement officer will be able to give specific advice on the careers and occupations open to the person with epilepsy, and those unsuitable such as driving a heavy goods vehicle or public service vehicle. He cannot hold a pilot's licence and must avoid machinery and heights, and possibly shift work. Employment rehabilitation centres may also give career guidance and provide training courses. The epilepsy association also runs a career assessment unit, giving advice about jobs and further education, and may do psychological assessments.

Leisure: Driving licences may be held if the individual has been free of fits for three years, or only has them at night. Leisure occupations must be sensible, heights and deep water being avoided, although swimming with someone competent to life-save can be indulged in. Children should be encouraged to join school camps and holidays. Alcohol will need to be restricted whilst the individual is on drugs. The epilepsy association can provide information about restrictions on travel or immigration.

Marriage: Genetic counselling must be given so that each individual can make an intelligent decision on whether to marry and have children or not. In most cases there is no contra-indication. If a woman with epilepsy becomes pregnant it is important that she is carefully controlled by drugs even though these may affect the baby.

Psychological factors: Although epilepsy may occur with brain damage, the majority of people with epilepsy are within the normal range of intelligence and there is no reason why they should not develop normally. However, where the condition is allowed to dominate the lives of those involved psychological problems may arise. Family relationships may be affected, with activities being restricted and other children becoming jealous.

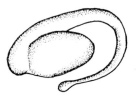 degeneration of
the basal ganglia

decreased production of
Dopamine

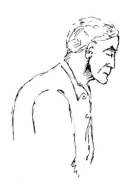
stooped   position
masklike features
shuffling gait
rigidity

pill rolling movement
of fingers
tremor of jaw and head
coarse tremor of limbs
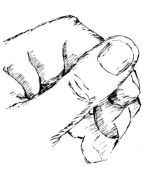

41 Parkinson's disease

PATHOLOGY

Parkinson's disease is a degenerative disorder of the basal nuclei. The pigmented cells of the basal nuclei form a chemical transmitter substance, **dopamine,** which travels to the corpus striatum to act as an inhibitor. The excitory transmitter substance is acetylcholine. These two substances normally balance one another. When degeneration of the basal nuclei occurs the amount of dopamine is decreased and therefore the balance is upset. As acetylcholine is now in excess the corpus striatum becomes over active causing the typical clinical picture. In the majority of cases the cause is unknown, but a similar condition can arise due to arteriosclerosis, and following encephalitis lethargica, manganese and carbon monoxide poisoning, head injury and very rarely after syphilis. Some drugs such as chlorporomazine, reserpine and haloperidol can also cause the same effects. Both men and women in their late middle years may be affected. The disease is characterised by poverty of movement, tremor and rigidity.

Poverty of movement
The ability to make facial expressions becomes less and less so that the patient is unable to smile, grimace or blink, and his face becomes masklike.

Tremor
There is a coarse tremor of the limbs which becomes less on movement. The tremor may also affect the lower jaw and head. The movements of the fingers may give the impression of pill rolling.

Increasing rigidity and inertia
There is a progressive stiffening of the limbs, the neck and shoulders becoming rigid, the individual stooping forward. Both initiating movement and stopping it become progressively more difficult, so that when rising out of a chair the patient appears like an automaton. If he walks he starts slowly, shuffling forward and then gradually increasing speed which he may be unable to control, and if he is pushed he will overbalance. When walking he does not swing his arms. Handwriting becomes very small and cramped. However, although he may look uninterested because of his lack of expression, his intellect remains unimpaired.

saliva may dribble
from the mouth
causing soreness of the chin

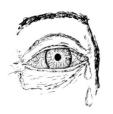

eyes may become
infected and painful
due to limited ability
to blink

be aware of the
problems caused by
reduced mobility and
difficulty in communication – it may
result in incontinence and a poor
dietary intake

It may be difficult to assess the patient's reactions because of his lack of facial expression, but it is important not to assume lack of mental awareness as these patients are usually mentally alert.

General appearance

The patient may appear undernourished because he has found it difficult to take in adequate nutrients. The nurse will need to find out whether the patient can feed himself, and if he can, how long it takes him. Is it so long that the meal becomes cold? His appetite may be impaired by drugs causing nausea, or he may have difficulty in chewing food. If there is drooling of saliva, this will cause embarrassment and soreness of the chin. There may be a limited ability to blink and as a result the eyes may become sore or infected.

Condition of the skin

Because of undernourishment pressure sores will develop if the patient is confined to bed, and therefore the areas at risk should be inspected.

Mental state

The patient has an alert mind behind his masklike face, and therefore he becomes rapidly frustrated. Relatives and friends may aggravate this if they are patronising. He may also be irritable with his relatives because of his forced dependence upon them, or because he feels they are deserting him.

Mobility

The nurse will need to find out exactly how much the patient can do for himself, and not take over activities he can still manage to do. Is he still mobile, and if so does he need assistance to go to the toilet or have a bath, or to wash and dress himself?

Excretion

Incontinence may occur either due to reduced mobility or because of difficulties in communication. Retention of urine and constipation may be present as a result of the disease or as a side effect of one of the drugs.

Communication

The difficulties which the patient may have in communication will need to be assessed carefully to see if he can say what he wants, or whether it is so slow and mumbled that it is difficult to understand.

155

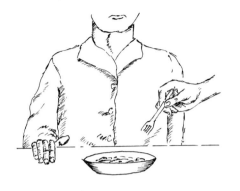

assist the patient
with feeding to ensure
an adequate diet but
encouragement to be
independent is needed

good grooming and
cleanliness is to be an
important step in his
rehabilitation – but
assistance may be needed
to avoid exhaustion

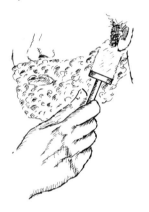

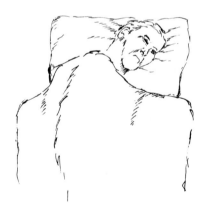

care of the patient
confined to bed will
include frequent
changes of position

If the nursing care plan is discussed with the patient and his relatives, the latter can be involved in ways which are most helpful to the patient, and this will help him feel that they have not deserted him.

Care of the skin
Allow the patient to do as much as he is able to do for himself but don't allow him to become exhausted or frustrated. He may need some help with cleaning his teeth and shaving. If confined to bed a sheepskin may be the best preventive measure against pressure sores, combined with frequent changes of position.

Nutrition
Discussion with the patient will ensure that a satisfactory compromise is reached between adequate nutrition and as much independence as possible. If he is able to feed himself but takes a long time, it may be better for the nurse or relative to feed him at the main meal of the day, and for the patient to manage on his own at the other meals. Special cutlery and crockery may help. A fluid balance chart should be kept to watch that an adequate intake of fluids is being taken. If there is any nausea or vomiting due to drugs such as L-dopa an antiemetic will be required.

Psychological care
Both the patient and the nurses will need to be very tolerant. Recognition of the reason why the patient is frustrated will help, but he also needs positive encouragement to make the most of the abilities he still has. Occasionally L-dopa causes mental disturbance, therefore any unusual behaviour should be reported.

Mobility
The patient should be encouraged to be up, and as independent as he is able, and will benefit from physiotherapy. He will be encouraged to lift his toes when walking, and to walk with his feet apart for balance. When he turns he should take a series of small steps and not cross his legs, this will help to prevent him falling over. A higher chair is better for sitting as it is easier to get out of, his feet being supported by a stool. Various drugs will have been ordered by the doctor to reduce his rigidity and poverty of movement. L-dopa is converted to dopamine in the brain. It should be taken with meals and must not be given with a monoamineoxidase inhibitor. The dose is 250 mg a day increasing to the maximum dose tolerated. It is sometimes given (as Sinemet or Madopar) with an agent which prevents L-dopa being converted to dopamine in the systemic circulation and thereby producing side effects such as nausea and vomiting, cardiac arrythmias, postural hypotension, fainting, further involuntary movements, mental disturbance and

constipation is to be
avoided and
may require
aperients or
suppositories

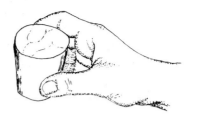

observations are required
to monitor side effects of
the patient's treatment

observations should also include
VISION for blurred sight or infection
SPEECH where therapy will assist
the patient's recovery

overactivity. Anticholinergic drugs such as benzhexol hydrochloride (Artane) 6–10 mg or orphenadrine hydrochloride (Disipal) 50–150 mg may be given and these may cause a dry mouth, blurred vision, constipation and urinary retention. Amantadine, an antiviral agent, is sometimes used. In some patients destruction of a small area of cells in the basal ganglia is done by stereotactic thalomotomy. Cryosurgery (freezing), or thermocoagulation may be performed on a small artery supplying that part of the basal ganglia. Afterwards there may be a transient hemiplegia, confusion or loss of temperature control. Unlike drug therapy this treatment appears to control the tremor.

Continence
If the patient is up he may need assistance in walking to the toilet, and in particular, aid in getting out of a chair and off the toilet. Regular toileting is necessary whether the patient is up or in bed. Output must be watched as anticholinergic drugs can cause urinary retention. If there is any constipation aperients or suppositories may be required.

Communication
Speech therapy will be started to help improve the patients ability to communicate. Practice with tongue twisters helps.

Special senses
Blurred vision arising from drug therapy will interfere with reading and other activities requiring good sight, and he may therefore appreciate someone reading to him. He should be taught to blink his eyes regularly to protect the surface of his eyes and if there is any infection the appropriate drops or ointment will have be prescribed.

Observations
These are mainly necessary because of the drugs being used. The pulse will be regularly checked for irregularities as cardiac arrythmias may occur if L-dopa is being taken. Postural hypotension is another side effect of this drug, therefore four-hourly blood pressure readings will also be taken. Chest infections frequently occur and early recognition and treatment is important, so the temperature will also be monitored carefully.

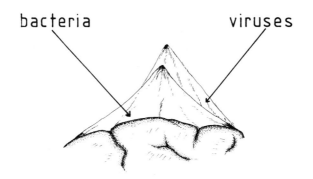

bacteria   viruses

infective   organisms   include :-

meningococcus. pneumococcus. staphylococcus
haemophilus influenzae   mycobacterium (T.B.)

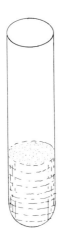

diagnosis is confirmed   by

1. lumbar puncture
2. blood culture

MENINGITIS

42 Meningitis

PATHOLOGY

Meningitis is inflammation of the meninges due to the invasion of micro-organisms. These organisms may be bacteria or viruses. The meningococcus, pneumococcus and haemolytic streptococcus are all pyogenic bacteria capable of causing meningitis. In the newborn baby, *E.Coli* and *Staphylococcus* may also be a cause, and in children *Haemophilus influenzae* (which does not cause influenza). The tubercle bacillus causes tuberculous meningitis. Viruses causing other illnesses such as mumps, polio, and measles can also cause meningitis. Bacterial meningitis can occur spontaneously, or be secondary to other infections such as otitis media, sinusitis, mastoiditis and septicaemia, as well as meningomyelocele, or fracture of the skull. Diagnosis is by means of a lumbar puncture and blood cultures.

CSF findings in meningitis

	Normal	*Bacterial*	*Viral*	*Tuberculous*
Colour	clear	cloudy or purulent	clear	clear
Sugar	normal	low	normal	low
Protein	normal	normal	raised	raised
Cells	nil	polymorphs	lymphocytes	lymphocytes

Inflammation of the meninges causes cerebral irritation and evidence of raised intracranial pressure. Neck stiffness is present, and the rigidity may be severe enough for the back to be arched and the head extended. Inflammation of the meninges covering the spinal cord causes sensitivity to any stretching as would happen if the hips are flexed and the legs straightened (**Kernig's sign**), which will therefore be resisted.

NURSING ASSESSMENT

Meningitis occurs most commonly in children and can be fatal, particularly if the child's resistance is already lowered due to previous infection.

General appearance
The child lies quietly in bed, turned away from the light and afraid to move. The way in which he lies and his lack of interest in what is happening around him indicate how ill he is. He may have a grey or pale look. In an infant the fontanelle should be observed as it may be bulging which indicates a raised intracranial pressure, or depressed showing dehydration. With certain types of meningitis a

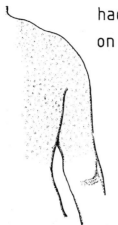

haemorrhagic rash may develop
on trunk and limbs

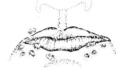

herpes around the
lips may be seen

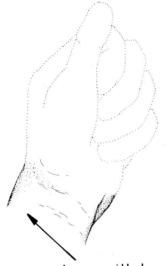

pulse will be slow

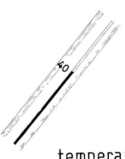

temperature will
be raised

haemorrhagic rash occurs which must be watched for, and herpes may arise around the lips. In an infant or small child dehydration frequently occurs and therefore evidence of this such as sunken eyes, inelastic skin, and depressed fontanelle will be noted. The patient will not want to eat or take feeds and may also be vomiting which will add to the dehydration.

Mental state
The patient may be merely drowsy, but may become stuporous or even comatose. If he is conscious there will be restlessness and irritability and a high pitched cry may be noted.

Mobility
He will not want to move or be moved and may be unconscious. Any attempt to straighten and lift the legs will be resisted. His neck will also be rigid and in severe cases the back may be arched and the neck extended.

Excretion
With dehydration being present there is likely to be constipation and a diminished urinary output. If the patient is unconscious then incontinence will also be present.

Special senses
There is usually an inability to tolerate light and therefore the patient will turn his head away from it (**photophobia**). It is important at all stages of the child's progress through the disease to note if there appears to be any difficulty in hearing or sight as either of these senses can be affected by the condition or sometimes by the treatment. Any evidence of otitis media or sinusitis may reveal where the infection originated.

Observations
The temperature will probably be raised and there may be rigors; the pulse will be slow. In a child convulsions may occur.

NURSING CARE PLAN

The patient is isolated because of the infection, the latter being treated by an appropriate antibiotic such as penicillin, chloramphenicol or sulphonamides, or antituberculous drugs in the case of tuberculous meningitis. If acutely ill steroids may be given. Where there is a source of infection such as otitis media this also will be treated. Sedatives will also be required.

Care of the skin
Frequent washes or even tepid sponging will be necessary if the temperature is raised and rigors occur. For the same reason, cotton

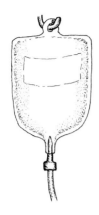

correct dehydration
correct electrolyte imbalance

record observations
accurately
report significant
changes

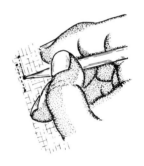

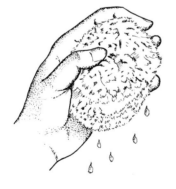

tepid sponging if
rigors occur
frequent skin care
regular turning

nightwear will be more comfortable than nylon. Two-hourly turning will be essential to prevent pressure sores and chest complications, but this must be done very gently as any movement is distressing to the patient. A ripple bed may be helpful in preventing pressure sores. If the patient is unconscious then the usual care of the mouth and eyes will be necessary. If conscious, frequent mouthwashes and sharp tasting substances can be used to stimulate the flow of saliva and keep the mouth fresh.

Nutrition
Any dehydration will need to be corrected, bearing in mind that the patient will lose even more fluid due to his pyrexia. Fluids will therefore be encouraged, iced drinks helping to reduce the patient's temperature. However if he is unconscious or unable to take sufficient fluids orally an intravenous infusion will be commenced by the doctor. This will also be used to correct any electrolyte disturbance. The nurse will carry out all the relevant observations. If nutrients are not being taken orally, a nasogastric tube may be passed and sufficient calories and nutrients given this way. As the patient's condition improves the intravenous infusion and nasogastric tube will be removed and a light diet introduced.

Psychological care
Once the patient has recovered consciousness and recovery is taking place the mental state will need to be assessed as mental retardation may occur as a complication.

Mobility
If unconscious, nursing will be as for any other unconscious patient. He will be kept in bed until the temperature is down and the general condition is improved.

Continence
Constipation frequently occurs and may need suppositories to correct it. The fluid balance must be carefully monitored because urinary retention may occur.

Special senses
The patient will be nursed in a darkened room because of the photophobia. Any evidence of deafness or blindness must still be watched for.

Observations
Four-hourly temperature, pulse, and respiration should be recorded, together with neurological observations, particularly alterations in level of consciousness. Note any cough or other evidence of chest infection and any change in colour particularly if he becomes grey and drawn looking. In an infant the size of the head will be measured daily for evidence of enlarging which would indicate a hydrocephalus. Nose and throat swabs may be taken.

165

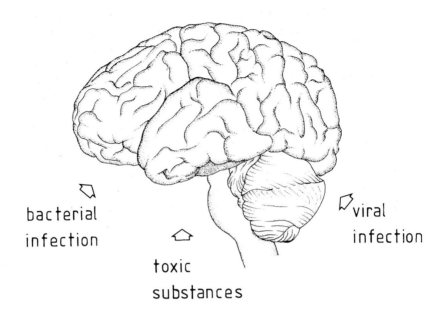

bacterial
infection

toxic
substances

viral
infection

disturbance of co-ordination
and movement

spasticity of limbs

fits

diagnosis

blood
specimen

stool and throat
swabs

lumbar
puncture

43 Encephalitis

Encephalitis is a severe, diffuse inflammation of the brain, and arises as a result of bacterial or viral infection. The latter is usually following a generalised disease such as measles, polio or pneumonia. The virus herpes simplex which causes the cold sore commonly found on the lips has also been found to cause encephalitis. In the very young it may be rapidly fatal, and in the adult produces an acute illness, which also may have a fatal outcome. The clinical picture may be very similar to that of meningitis. If the motor areas of the brain are involved then co-ordination and movement will be upset and there may be spasticity of the limbs. The pattern of sleep may also be altered, and fits are often a prominent feature. Diagnosis is by lumbar puncture although the results may not be known for some time. A throat swab and specimens of blood and faeces will also be taken. Treatment is symptomatic and therefore nursing care is of prime importance, being similar to that in meningitis.

Circle of Willis

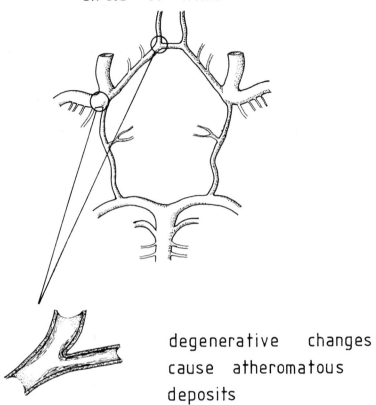

degenerative changes
cause atheromatous
deposits

increasing   blood   pressure

aneurysm occurs at
the weak point

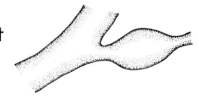

44 Subarachnoid haemorrhage

PATHOLOGY

It is thought that in many people there is a congenital weakness in the walls of the larger cerebral blood vessels where they join one another in the circle of Willis. As the individual grows older, degenerative changes occur, atheroma is deposited and the blood pressure increases. As a result, ballooning occurs at these weak points so forming an aneurysm. There may be more than one aneurysm present, the majority being found in the anterior half of the circle of Willis. These aneurysms usually occur when the individual is forty or fifty, although they may be present earlier. More women than men appear to be affected.

Sometimes the aneurysm becomes large enough to press on a nearby structure and cause symptoms. There maybe interference in the function of the pituitary or one of the cranial nerves. If the third cranial nerve is affected there will be drooping of the eylid (**ptosis**), and double vision. Pressure on the second cranial nerve will cause the visual fields to be affected, and occasionally blindness. Pressure on the fifth cranial nerve will result in pain or numbness of the face and even facial palsy.

Increase in the blood pressure from exertion, bending over, or a severe bout of coughing may eventually be sufficient to rupture one of these aneurysms causing bleeding into the subarachnoid space. This is what normally happens if the aneurysm is small. If, however, the aneurysm enlarges it may burrow into the substance of the brain when rupture of it will cause bleeding into the brain itself and a similar outcome to a cerebrovascular accident.

The diagnosis is made by lumbar puncture, in which the cerebrospinal fluid is uniformly blood stained. If the specimen is allowed to stand the fluid has a yellowish tinge (xanthochromic). The pressure will also be raised. With conservative treatment the following outcome is to be expected:

40–50% die within eight weeks
10% die before six months
10% die at some later date
Of the 30% who survive:
1/3 are symptom free

169

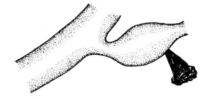

coughing, bending or exertion may cause an increase in blood pressure and rupture of the aneurysm

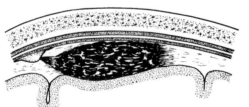

resulting in bleeding into the subarachnoid space

⅓ have severe neurological symptoms such as:
   epileptiform fits
   headaches
   hemiparesis
   psychological disturbance
⅓ have less severe symptoms

Some doctors prescribe epsilon aminocaproic acid in the hope that this will reduce further bleeding.

When the patient's condition has improved and he has regained consciousness surgery may be considered if the neurological changes are minimal. This will depend not only on his general condition but also on his age. Surgery is less likely to be performed in patients over fifty. The actual site and size of the aneurysm will also be an important deciding factor. If there is a generalised vascular disorder this will also be a contraindication for an operation.

Operative procedures

A metal clip may be put across the neck of the aneurysm. The aneurysm may be wrapped around with muscle, connective tissue from the leg, or substances such as muslin or acrylic. Sometimes the internal carotid artery in the neck is tied off to reduce the pressure in the aneurysm fed by it. The operation may be done under deep hypothermia which will be maintained for thirty six hours after the operation.

observations will show
a raised blood pressure

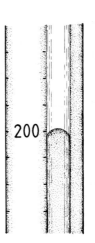

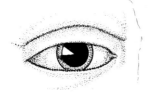

dilation of the pupil
& disturbance of
vision

headache
neck stiffness
photophobia

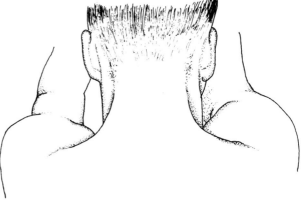

This condition may occur suddenly without warning in what otherwise may appear to be a healthy middle aged adult.

General appearance
The patient will probably be lying very still, and turned away from the light. He will complain of a severe headache which is either in the frontal or occipital region to start with but later becomes more generalised. Vomiting is frequently present. There will almost certainly be neck stiffness. If the facial nerve is affected there may be numbness in the face or even paralysis.

Mental state
Drowsiness or confusion is usually present although the patient may be restless and irritable. Occasionally the patient becomes rapidly unconscious.

Mobility
Although not usual, occasionally a patient may develop hemiparesis or a hemiplegia.

Special senses
There is often disturbed vision due to haemorrhage from the blood vessels in the retina, and there may be double vision if the optic nerve is affected. In some patients blindness occurs.

Observations
There is some degree of raised intracranial pressure and the blood pressure will be raised accordingly. Compression of the third cranial nerve, if present, will cause dilatation of the pupil. In some patients epileptiform fits occur.

a light diet - easily digested
assistance with feeding
straws used for drinking

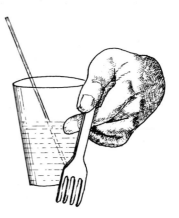

ANALGESICS
at the correct time

SEDATION
night and/or day

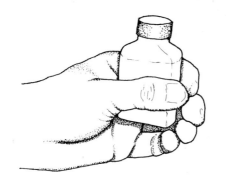

ANTI-EMETIC
to prevent patient
vomiting

monitor patient's blood pressure

If the patient is unconscious he should be cared for as described in Chapter 34.

Care of the skin

Bedbaths and pressure area care will need to be carried out with the minimum of movement and therefore a sheepskin or ripple bed may be of particular benefit. As the patient may be vomiting, oral care will be important, the nurse gently cleaning the teeth with a tooth brush and allowing the patient to rinse his mouth with a mouth wash.

Nutrition

The patient will be lying flat so he will need a light diet which is easily digested. Initially he will have to be fed although he may use a plastic straw for fluids. Any antiemetics prescribed should be given to prevent the patient vomiting, not waiting until he does so.

Psychological care

Quietness is important so visitors will be restricted, although they may help by reading to the patient or even feeding him, if he is agreeable. The nurse will be responsible for seeing that a sufficient-ly strong analgesic has been written up, and that the patient is not kept waiting for it. Sedation wll also be given.

Mobility

Patient's are nursed in a quiet dark room and will remain on bed-rest for six weeks. They should not be moved unnecessarily, but nursed in the position most comfortable to them. However such management will mean that they are particularly at risk for devel-oping chest infections and deep vein thrombosis. Therefore the physiotherapist will give passive exercises and encourage deep breathing, which the nurses will continue. After six weeks if the patient is not having surgery he will be carefully mobilised.

Continence

A slipper bedpan may be more comfortable as the patient will have to remain flat. Two nurses should lift him onto the bedpan. Because of the difficulty of defaecation on a bedpan, regular aperients will be given to avoid constipation and straining.

Special senses

The nurse or relatives may help the patient by reading to him.

Observations

The blood pressure, temperature, pulse, and respiration will be taken four hourly, unless the patient's condition requires more fre-quent observation. The strength of the patient's grip may also be tested regularly. Neurological observations will be very import-ant. Occasionally a mild hypotensive drug is given, another reason for monitoring the blood pressure.

175

lesions at this
point result in
quadriplegia and
respiratory paralysis

lesions are not
compatible with
life above this
point

lesions at this
point result in
disturbance of
bowel and bladder
reflex and sexual
function

in syringomyelia
the centre of the
cord is affected

45 Lesions of the spinal cord

The spinal cord may damaged by trauma in the form of penetrating wounds or a whip-lash injury, or it may be affected by disease, tumours or an abscess. The effects of trauma depend on the severity of the lesion and the level at which it occurs. Trauma which does not sever the spinal cord but causes 'concussion' of it, will initially cause the same effects as if it had been severed, but these effects will rapidly wear off. Tumours usually occur outside the spinal cord and cause damage by pressing on it. Metastasis can occur from any other site in the body. The clinical picture will be according to the level of the lesion and the speed at which it grows. Although the tumour may be removed, irreparable damage may occur as a result of the operation. Radiotherapy may sometimes be effective.

The higher the level at which the lesion occurs the greater the effects. A lesion above the level of the fourth cervical vertebra is incompatible with life. Just below this level there will be complete quadriplegia and paralysis of the respiratory muscles necessitating the patient being on a ventilator. Lesions in the lumbar region will cause a paraplegia with interference in the reflex emptying of the bladder and bowel, and sexual function. Damage to one half of the spinal cord will cause paralysis on that side below the level of the lesion and loss of proprioception, on that side, but loss of pain and temperature sensation on the other side. (Brown-Séquard syndrome). In syringomyelia the centre of the spinal cord is affected causing damage to the sensory fibres that cross over at that point so causing loss of sensation at one level only.

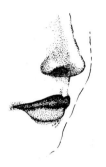

the virus enters nasopharynx
or mouth. if the organism is
not destroyed it enters the
BLOODSTREAM

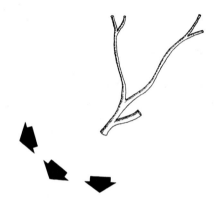

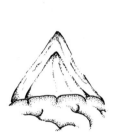

meninges

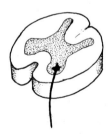

anterior horn cells
of the spinal cord

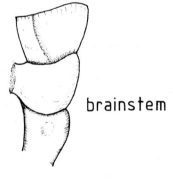

brainstem

46 Anterior poliomyelitis

PATHOLOGY

Anterior poliomyelitis is a notifiable infectious disease affecting children and young adults. There are three different viruses causing the disease, each of which is capable of causing paralysis. Although they all stimulate the production of antibodies, the immunity acquired to one form does not give protection against the other two. It appears to be a common viral infection spread by faecal contamination of food and water and communal places such as swimming baths, particularly in areas where the hygiene is poor. In such an environment the very young may contract the disease without being ill, so developing a lasting immunity. The older the individual when the disease is contracted the more likely paralysis is to develop.

The virus enters the body via the nasopharynx and the gastro-intestinal tract where it multiplies. If the infection is virulent, or the antibodies insufficient to destroy the viruses, they pass into the blood stream and from there to other tissues such as the meninges, and anterior horn cells in the spinal cord and the brain stem. Within the nervous tissue the viruses multiply until eventually the nerve cells are destroyed, and therefore the muscles supplied by those nerves become paralysed. When it affects the motor cell bodies in the spinal cord this is a lower motor neurone disease. If the virus attacks the spinal cord one or more limbs may be affected according to the level which is affected. **Bulbar poliomyelitis** damages the cranial nerve cells in the brain stem, particularly affecting facial (VII), palatal and pharyngeal (IX), and eye movements (VI and III), and the vagus (larynx, respiration and heart) (X). Bulbospinal poliomyelitis combines both forms.

As there is no specific treatment for the condition it is obviously better to prevent it occurring at all, and this can be done by giving a vaccine to those susceptible in the community. Originally the **Salk** vaccine developed in the 1950's was used. This utilises killed viruses, but because of this the immunity does not last and booster doses have to be given. In the early 1960's the **Sabin** oral vaccine was developed. In this preparation live, weakened viruses are used and therefore the immune response will last much longer. Three doses are usually needed, and they contain the three viruses. Booster doses are necessary in epidemics or when travelling to high-risk areas. In an outbreak the vaccine is given to those in contact. Young people in particular are advised to avoid crowds and especially swimming baths. Over exertion should also be avoided. Control of flies and care in the disposal of sewage is also important, as well as a high standard of hygiene amongst those

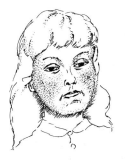

NON PARALYTIC
DISEASE

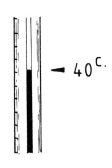

$40^C.$

flushed and
apathetic

slightly raised
temperature

difficulty in breathing
and swallowing

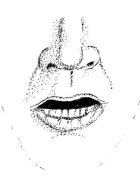

PARALYTIC DISEASE

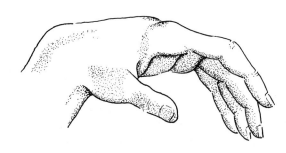

paralysis of affected
limbs

handling food. Minor operations such as tonsillectomies and dental extractions are best postponed.

In this way contact with the virus is less likely, and the resistance of those at risk is not unnecessarily lowered.

NURSING ASSESSMENT

The nurse may encounter the patient at any one of the stages of this condition, each of which will require different care.

Non-paralytic disease

General appearance: The patient, who is usually a child or young adult, appears flushed and generally disinclined to do anything. If movement is attempted there may be some stiffness in the back, legs and neck as with meningitis. The patient may complain of a headache and the temperature may also be slightly raised. Nausea or even vomiting may make the patient disinclined to eat, and added to this, if he has a sore throat, he may also find difficulty in swallowing. This state may last two to four days and then clear up completely, or after 48 hours develop into the paralytic form. It is therefore important for the nurse to observe carefully for early signs.

Paralytic disease

Mental state: The patient will obviously be distressed at the progressive nature of the condition, fearing complete paralysis.

Mobility: Flaccid paralysis may affect one or more limbs but more commonly affects the lower limbs. Because it is a lower motor neurone disease the reflexes are also absent and the muscles involved waste. These muscles may be very tender with muscle spasm in the early stages.

Excretion: Retention of urine and constipation are common and should therefore be watched for.

Observations: Any tendency to talk in short staccato sentences or a weakening of the voice indicates that the patient is having some difficulty in breathing. This is particularly likely to happen when the spinal lesion is high involving the arms, diaphragm, and intercostal muscles. If it is not recognised early enough it will lead on to respiratory failure. Should the patient start to regurgitate fluids through the nose or have difficulty in swallowing this indicates paralysis of the palate and pharynx, which again could be fatal. If the vagus is involved there may be a rattle of secretions at the back of the throat when breathing, which on inspection can be seen as frothy secretions at the back of the throat, or slight choking attacks may occur.

181

REST – in a comfortable position
ISOLATION – to prevent spread

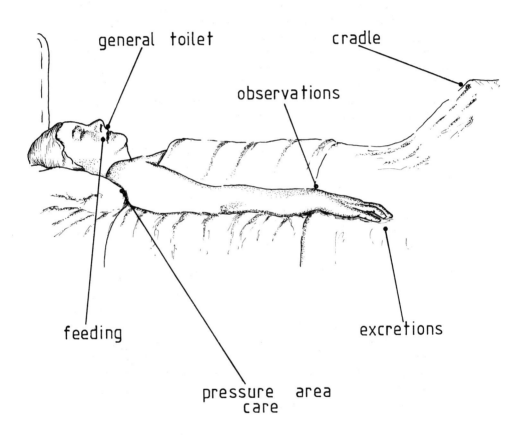

general toilet

cradle

observations

feeding

excretions

pressure area
care

General appearance: If the brain stem is affected there may be paralysis of the facial muscles squinting and double vision. Photophobia may also be present.

NURSING CARE PLAN

Non-paralytic disease

These patients are usually nursed in special units to prevent spread of the condition to others through faecal contamination. They, themselves, also require protection from other infections.

General care of the skin: Gentle washing, sufficient to keep the patient comfortable, will be necessary if the patient is perspiring. For the same reason cotton night-clothes may be more comfortable. The patient will probably prefer to clean his own teeth and use a mouth wash. Movement can be very painful, so unnecessary movement should be avoided, but when it is done, may be less painful if two or three nurses do it together. Massage of vulnerable areas may be too distressing to the patient and should therefore be avoided. Therefore two hourly turning will be of major importance and a sheepskin or large cell ripple bed may be the best aids.

Nutrition: Fluids must be encouraged unless there is any difficulty in swallowing, in which case semisolids are tolerated better than fluids or solids.

Psychological care: This patient will need all the support he can get from the medical and nursing staff to allay his fears. Honesty about the progress of the disease is essential.

Mobility: The bed should have a firm base, but is more comfortable for the patient if the mattress is soft. The most comfortable position for the patient is usually recumbent. Not only does he need rest generally for his body, but the muscles affected must be rested in an effort to prevent paralysis occurring. A cradle is useful in keeping heavy bedclothes off painful limbs. The latter should be positioned carefully, not putting any strain on the joints. Passive movements may be done if they are not too painful. If there is any muscle spasm then hot packs may relieve this.

Continence: Urinary output must be monitored very carefully by means of a fluid balance chart. If constipation is present, suppositories will be required and a regular check of bowel motions made. Abdominal distension may be relieved by a flatus tube, or prostigmine.

Observations: Four hourly temperature, pulse and respiration should be recorded unless abnormality in the respirations require

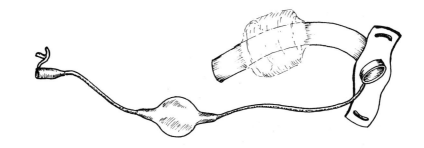

CUFFED TRACHEOSTOMY

to avoid fluid entering
the lungs.
to aspirate the lungs.
to assist ventilation.

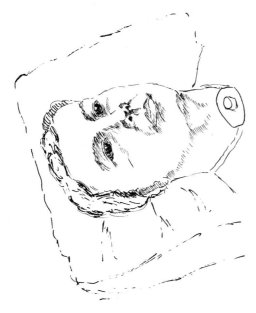

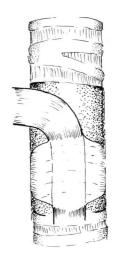

more frequent observation. If there is any weakness of the limbs the vital capacity will be checked twice daily with a spirometer.

Paralytic disease

Care of the skin: This will be as before, but oral hygiene will be particularly important.

Nutrition: The patient will be fed with a fine naso-gastric tube or possibly a gastrostomy tube.

Psychological care: This will be of even greater importance, as the patient will be completely dependent on the medical and nursing staff for his needs. His relatives also will need support.

Continence: If urinary retention is not relieved by drugs, catheterisation will be necessary. Therefore catheter toilet and changing of the urinary drainage bag will need to be attended to.

Maintenance of efficient respiration: Damage in the medulla will cause difficulty in swallowing with danger of fluid being aspirated. The patient will therefore need to be in a head-down position, with a cuffed tracheostomy tube and regular aspiration. Postural drainage will also assist the removal of secretions from the lungs. If respiration is inadequate, for whatever reason, a tracheostomy will be performed with assisted ventilation. In patients where respiratory failure persists the tank respirator or the cuirasse respirator will be used.

In the recovery phase
Physiotherapy aims at recovering as much movement as possible in the limbs. A realistic but positive outlook is essential. Orthopaedic operations may be necessary if there is any resulting deformity interfering with function.

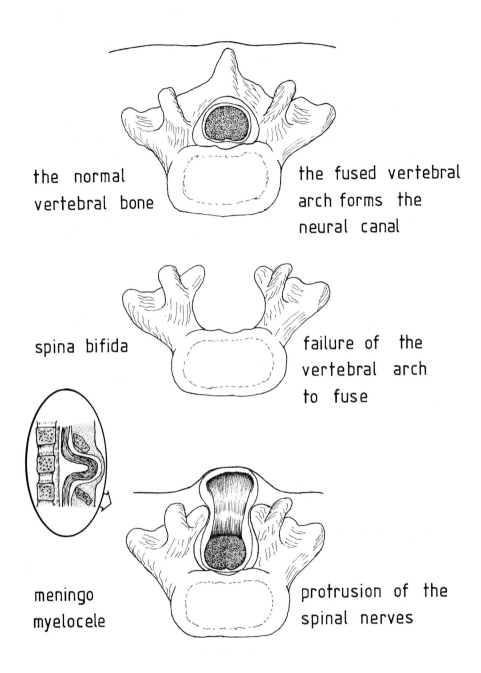

the normal
vertebral bone

the fused vertebral
arch forms the
neural canal

spina bifida

failure of the
vertebral arch
to fuse

meningo
myelocele

protrusion of the
spinal nerves

47 Spina bifida

This condition arises due to an abnormality in the development of the vertebral column. The spinal processes do not fuse together to form the neural arch. It most commonly occurs in the lumbar region but can be anywhere in the vertebral column.

Spina bifida occulta

In this condition there is non-fusion of the vertebrae but the meninges and the nervous tissue are not involved. There may be a naevus, dimple, or hair over the affected area, and because no nervous tissue is involved there are no problems. It is probably a common condition although the incidence is not known.

Meningocele

In this case the meninges prolapse through the bony defect. It is not a very common condition and with treatment there are not usually complications.

Meningomyelocele or spina bifida cystica

More common than the meningocele, this involves prolapse of the cord and the meninges, with stretching of the spinal nerves. Because the latter contain both motor and sensory nerves there is a paralysis of the parts supplied and loss of sensation leading to ulceration of the skin. It is associated with urinary incontinence and repeated urinary infections which can eventually lead to progressive renal failure. The joints may be either lax or spastic. The nerve supply to some of the muscles may be intact although their antagonists are paralysed, which will cause severe flexion often at the hips resulting in dislocation or fractures. Spina bifida is associated with other deformities such as kyphosis, lordosis, scoliosis of the spine or talipes of the feet, and hydrocephalus.

It is possible to detect the condition whilst the fetus is developing *in utero*, at sixteen to eighteen weeks, by doing an **amniocentesis**. From tests on the amniotic fluid, abnormal levels of **alpha-fetoprotein** can be detected. This is a test which is only carried out on those women at risk, for example if the woman has already had a baby with a spina bifida, or there is a history of it in the family. Eventually a reliable serum test may be developed which can be used as a screening device for all pregnant women.

MANAGEMENT

Those babies who have not already got extensive abnormalities and have a good chance of benefiting will be selected for surgery. This is carried out within 24 hours of birth under antibiotic cover.

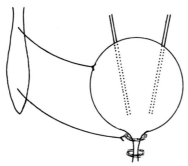

nerves controlling
the bladder and
sphincters arise
in the lumbar and sacral segments of
the spinal cord

spina bifida may result in loss of
nerve control and urinary incontinence-
ileal conduit
surgery may be
necessary

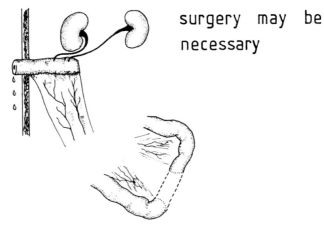

The exposed nervous tissue is covered with dura mater and skin. Postoperatively the infant is handled as little as possible, observing in particular the urinary output and any signs of developing meningitis or hydrocephalus. It will be nursed prone in an incubator to maintain warmth. Tube feeding may be necessary in the early stages. Care is taken to prevent pressure sores developing. Urinary incontinence in boys may be controlled by collecting devices, but in the majority of girls and some boys an ileal conduit may be necessary before the child starts school. Urinary infections will be a constant problem and may lead to progressive renal failure.

Orthopaedic operations will be required to correct any deformities of the lower limbs and muscles may be transplanted. For example the ilio-psoas muscle may be taken through the ilium of the pelvis into the back of the greater trochanter to act as an extensor and abductor of the hip in opposition to the remaining flexors and adductors, so giving some degree of stability to the hip joint.

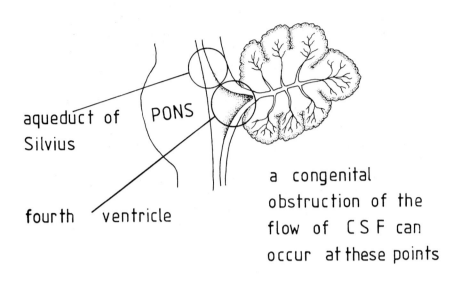

aqueduct of Silvius

PONS

fourth ventricle

a congenital obstruction of the flow of CSF can occur at these points

unrelieved ventricular pressure of CSF results in tissue destruction and brain damage

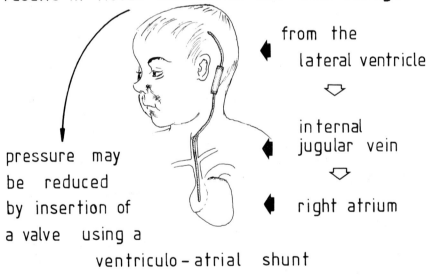

from the lateral ventricle

internal jugular vein

right atrium

pressure may be reduced by insertion of a valve using a ventriculo–atrial shunt

48 Hydrocephalus

Hydrocephalus occurs as a result of deficient absorption of the cerebrospinal fluid. Obstruction in the exit from the fourth ventricle into the subarachnoid space is the most common reason. This may be present at birth, in which case there may be other associated congenital defects such as spina bifida, or it may result from meningitis or occasionally a brain tumour. Because absorption is less than secretion there is an increase in the amount of cerebrospinal fluid circulating and therefore increased intracranial pressure.

In an infant the skull bones are not ossified, and therefore as the amount of cerebrospinal fluid increases the head enlarges. If untreated the cranial part of the head looks too large for the face, the forehead bulging. The increased intracranial pressure causes the fontanelles to enlarge and become distended and tense, and the scalp veins to be engorged. Because of the pressure the eyes look down, giving the appearance of the 'setting sun'. Increasing cerebrospinal fluid in the ventricles means that the head can easily be transilluminated. Gradually the brain will become progressively more damaged although there may be a spontaneous arrest of the condition at any stage. Severe brain damage will mean that the child may be unable to do anything for itself and may be blind or deaf. Pressure on the vital centres in the medulla oblongata will lead to death.

In order to differentiate between hydrocephalus and other disorders which may cause raised intracranial pressure, a ventricular tap will be done. An air ventriculogram or a dye test may also be used to check whether there is any drainage from the ventricles into the subarachnoid space. Treatment is aimed at providing a means of draining the cerebrospinal fluid from the ventricles into the venous system. The surgeon makes an incision behind the right ear into which he introduces a one-way valve. A length of silicone rubber tubing is passed through a burr hole into the lateral ventricle and connected to its upper end. Another piece of tubing links the valve to the internal jugular vein.

Several problems may arise once the valve is in position. Overdrainage will cause the fontanelle to become sunken, and this can be remedied by lowering the head and raising the feet. There may be insufficient drainage due to blockage, which will lead to increased intracranial pressure. This may be relieved by raising the head of the bed, milking the valve, and if this is insufficient, replacement of the valve. For this reason the tension of the fontanelle and the head circumference need to be monitored closely. Infection may enter via the valve causing a septicaemia and meningitis which will necessitate the valve being replaced, and the use of antibiotics. As the child grows so the tubing will need to be changed. The parents have to be taught how to pump the valve and recognise symptoms of raised intracranial pressure.

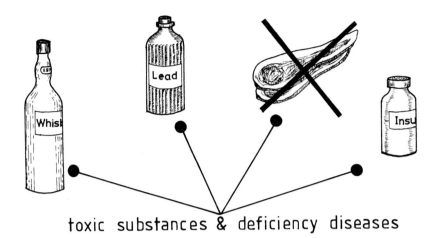

toxic substances & deficiency diseases

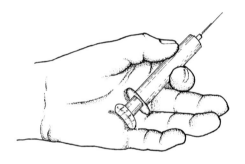

allergic response to
tetanus toxoid

lack of vitamin B_{12}
associated with
pernicious anaemia

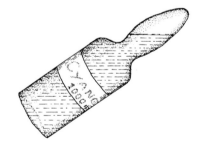

49　Peripheral neuritis

PATHOLOGY

Peripheral neuritis is really a group of different disorders affecting the peripheral nerves. The spinal nerves are the main ones to be affected although the cranial nerves may also be involved. The peripheral nerve cell, the myelin sheath, or the Schwann cell may be affected. These are mixed nerves and there is therefore a varying degree of disturbance in either sensory or motor function or both.

Subacute peripheral neuritis

Toxic substances and chemicals such as spirits, fortified wine, lead and arsenic may damage the lower motor neurone cell in the anterior horn of the spinal cord. Deficiency diseases, in particular lack of vitamin B1, and diabetes, may also have a similar effect. Although the damage is at cell level, degeneration will occur at the furthermost point of the nerve fibre, thus explaining why the symptoms start at the feet and work up the body.

In the alcoholic form there may be evidence of overdrinking with a furred tongue, florid complexion and shaking hands. The patient may also be undernourished and complaining of morning sickness and a poor appetite. He may also have an unsteady gait, or if badly affected may not even be able to walk. The arms may also be weak. This condition is associated with painful muscle cramps, the calves being very sensitive to pressure. Persistent retention of urine is also a feature. Depression, which can lead to alcoholism, may also be present, and dementia is associated with some chronic forms.

If peripheral neuritis is associated with diabetes this is usually because the latter is out of control. Treatment of the diabetes may improve the condition. If the condition is due to alcohol, the patient is advised to stop drinking and given vitamin B by injection. **Subacute combined degeneration** of the spinal cord is the result of vitamin B12 deficiency due to the lack of intrinsic factor in the stomach and is associated with pernicious anaemia.

Chronic peripheral neuritis

When the Schwann cells are affected the associated short segments of myelin sheath degenerate, (segmental demyelination). This occurs as a result of carcinoma, or for no known cause. The carcinoma frequently arises in the lungs although it may be elsewhere in the body, and the neuritis is not due to metastases but possibly to toxic effects.

Guillain-Barré syndrome—Acute polyneuritis

Inflammatory-allergic reactions sometimes related to viral infections such as mumps, herpes zoster or glandular fever, or an aller-

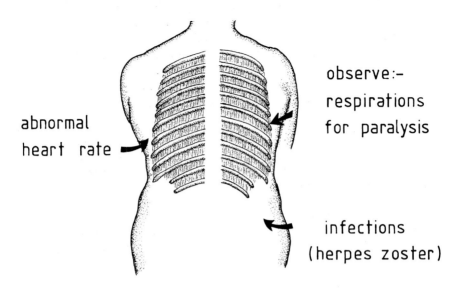

observe:-
respirations
for paralysis

abnormal
heart rate

infections
(herpes zoster)

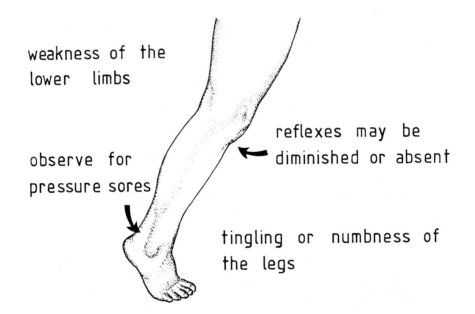

weakness of the
lower limbs

reflexes may be
diminished or absent

observe for
pressure sores

tingling or numbness of
the legs

gic response to tetanus toxoid, may cause demyelination of the peripheral nerves. This results in an acute polyneuritis which may be rapidly fatal, or else resolve completely within a relatively short time. It is this condition which is dealt with in the following pages. A lumbar puncture may be helpful in diagnosis as there is sometimes a significantly raised protein, although this is not always so.

ACUTE PERIPHERAL NEURITIS – NURSING ASSESSMENT

Whatever the cause of peripheral neuritis, the clinical picture has many factors in common. Acute polyneuritis develops rapidly, and is occasionally fatal, although there is usually complete recovery in a few weeks or months.

General appearance
The patient's underlying physical condition may be good because of the rapid onset of the disease, but he will obviously look acutely ill.

Condition of the skin
There is usually a tingling sensation which progresses to numbness in the legs. The skin needs to be examined carefully for any evidence of pressure sores because these are much more likely to occur in areas in which there is no sensation.

Mental state
The patient will be very frightened at the rapid progress of the condition, particularly if he starts to choke.

Mobility
Weakness of the lower limbs may gradually spread up the body to all limbs and the reflexes are diminished or absent.

Excretion
Although retention may occur it is usually temporary.

Special senses
The cranial nerves are much more likely to be affected in the acute form, particularly affecting swallowing.

Observations
There may be a history of an infection or this may still be evident, for example the skin lesions of herpes zoster may still be present. It will also be necessary to check if the patient has had tetanus serum recently. Respirations must be observed for any evidence of paralysis. The ability to swallow may also be affected so any evidence of choking must be noted as early as possible. A myocardial infarction may occur as a result of anoxia and therefore the heart rate must be checked for abnormalities which would indicate this.

195

catheter toilet and care of
urinary drainage

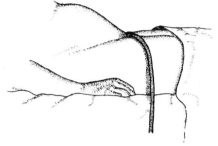

measure and record
fluid balance

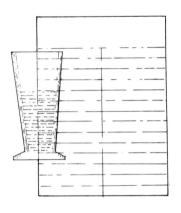

Antibiotics

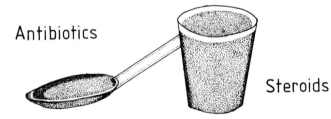

Steroids

Analgesics

The patient will be acutely ill and will need everything done for him. If respirations are inadequate, either intubation or tracheostomy may be required. In this case the nurse will have to carry out regular tracheal suction and care for the tracheostomy wound, bearing in mind that the patient will be unable to communicate and will therefore need special care.

Care of the skin
In areas where there is diminished sensation there is a high risk of pressure sores developing without the patient being aware of it, and therefore two-hourly turning and specific preventive care will be needed. The acutely ill patient will require the nurse to attend to his oral care at least four-hourly, particularly if nothing is being taken by mouth and suction is being used.

Nutrition
In the acute form intravenous feeding may be necessary in the initial stages, but will soon be replaced by intragastric feeding, preferably with a special narrow bore tube. Specially prepared feeds will be given to ensure adequate intake of the necessary nutrients and fluids.

Psychological care
The patient will be very distressed at his rapidly deteriorating condition in the early stages, and will therefore need the reassurance that he will recover. The relatives will also need this reassurance. Confidence in the nurse caring for him is vital, who must therefore know exactly what is required of her. She also needs to develop a sensitiveness to what he requires as his communication is limited. Once he is over the worst part, boredom will be pre-eminent as he is unable to do anything himself. Someone to read to him, a wireless, and a television may all help to alleviate boredom. Analgesics will have been prescribed by the doctor if pain is a prominent feature, and the nurse must recognise when these are required.

Mobility
In the acute stage passive physiotherapy will be carried out, putting all the joints through a full range of movements. Night splints may be necessary in the early stages to prevent foot and wrist drop. Eventually the patient will be able to do active exercises.

Continence
Whilst there is acute retention a catheter may be necessary, in which case the nurse will have to carry out the usual catheter toilet and care of the urinary drainage. If a catheter is not *in situ*, the patient must be carefully observed for any evidence of urinary

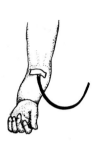

intravenous feeding
initially – followed
by intragastric
feeding

inadequate respirations may require a
tracheostomy

a tracheostomy requires
regular tracheal suction

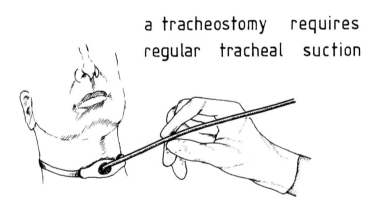

remember this is a   STERILE   technique

retention and resulting infection. Regularity of bowel motions should be aimed for.

Observations

While there is evidence of infection and danger of respiratory arrest the temperature, pulse and respiration, and the blood pressure, will be taken at least four-hourly. However, steroids, and especially ACTH, may given by the doctor as a specific form of treatment and may mask infection. Antibiotics may have been pre-scribed to prevent chest infection. If the patient has to be put on a ventilator the nurse will have to keep all the relevant observations. She will also watch for any evidence of electrolyte imbalance, such as increasing drowsiness, confusion or disturbed pulse rate. As the patient improves so these observations are decreased. The physio-therapist and the nurse will work together in taking the patient off the ventilator once the respiratory muscles are functioning.

trigeminal nerve
(fifth cranial)
divides into
three large
branches

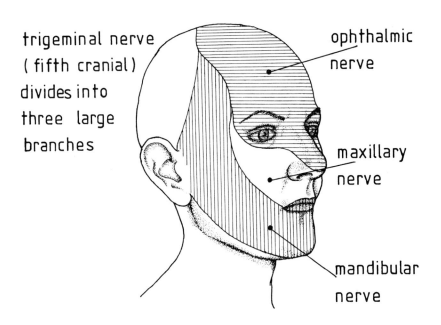

ophthalmic
nerve

maxillary
nerve

mandibular
nerve

facial nerve
(seventh cranial)
carries motor
fibres to
muscles of the
face

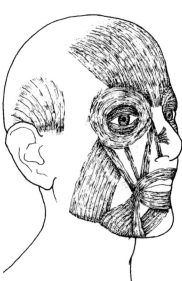

branches to
lacrimal glands
salivary glands
tongue (taste)

50 The trigeminal and facial nerves

Trigeminal neuralgia

The fifth cranial nerve (trigeminal) has three divisions supplying sensation to the head. The first division supplies the front two thirds of the scalp and part of the nose, the second division supplies cheeks, upper lips and nose, and the third division supplies the front of the lower jaw and the temporal area of the face. Trigeminal neuralgia occurs most commonly in women over the age of fifty, and usually affects one side of the face involving one or more branches of the trigeminal nerve, mainly the second or third. There is usually a trigger-point which is stimulated by a draught of cold air, touching when washing, shaving or eating, or movement in talking or eating. This triggers off a series of excruciating jabbing pains, which may last minutes or hours. The pain is so severe that the individual stops anything he is doing. The period between the attacks initially may be weeks or months. Gradually the attacks become longer, the periods between shorter, and the area affected greater. The cause of this condition is unknown, but it may be due to the protective myelin sheath being damaged by vascular changes, so enabling impulses to pass across from one fibre to another.

Anticonvulsant drugs such as phenytoin sodium (Epanutin) 400–500 mg daily or carbamezeprine (Tegretol) 200 mg daily, increasing to 1 g daily, may be given as treatment. There may be severe gastrointestinal side effects in which case the treatment may have to be stopped. An injection of alcohol into the nerve, or division of it, may relieve the pain, but result in anaesthesia of the area, and a burning sensation.

Bell's palsy

The seventh cranial nerve (facial) supplies the muscles of facial expression, and it also has some autonomic fibres which control the secretion of tears and saliva, and carries sensory fibres from the tongue (taste). This nerve may be damaged by pressure from a tumour or trauma. The cause of true Bell's palsy is unknown, although it may occur after herpes zoster. The nerve becomes unable to conduct nerve impulses so causing weakness or paralysis on the side of the face supplied by that nerve. The onset may be sudden or gradual. Because of the paralysis there is drooping of the mouth causing difficulty in eating and the patient is unable to close the eye. Spontaneous recovery usually occurs.

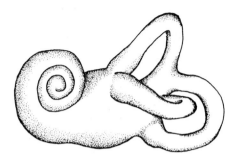

CAUSE

an increase in the pressure of endolymph
in the labyrinth and cochlear of the
inner ear

giddiness and loss of balance
nausea, vomiting, prostration and shock
nystagmus, tinnitus and deafness

anti-emetic drugs
    help to control vomiting

sedatives
    reduce number of attacks

51 Menières disease

This condition arises as a result of an intermittent increase in the endolymph which fills the labyrinth and the cochlea of the ear and damages the receptors in these two organs. Why it occurs is unknown but it may be due to some vascular disturbance. Gradually the receptor organs are destroyed.

The patient will suffer from sudden, severe attacks of giddiness, such that he feels that everything is whirling around him, or that he is spinning in an uncontrollable manner. Any movement aggravates the situation. It may be so bad that he falls to the ground. It is always associated with nausea, and often with uncontrollable vomiting, prostration and shock. There may even be incontinence due to loss of sphincter control. Nystagmus, rapid movements of the eyes, is also present. Most patients with Menières disease have noises in the ear (**tinnitus**) which may become worse just before an attack of vertigo begins. There is progressive deafness, at first in one ear but eventually affecting both sides, which is more marked for noise at a low intensity, loud tones being heard normally. There may also be a full feeling in the affected ear. The attacks can last from thirty minutes to several hours, and may occur several times within the week, but there may be months between them. As the receptor organs are progressively destroyed on one side the attacks become less disturbing, although as the other side becomes affected they may increase again for a while.

Audiometry will be done to assess the level of hearing, and caloric tests to assess the function of the semicircular canals and the vestibular apparatus.

This is a very distressing condition for the patient, and he will need a full explanation of what is happening and how the condition is expected to progress. If his work involves climbing ladders he will be advised to find something he can do from ground level. Antiemetic drugs such as chlorpromazine, Dramamine, or Avomine may help to control the vomiting and should be taken at the first sign of an impending attack. Sedatives taken on a regular basis may help to reduce the number of attacks. If the disease affects one side only and is causing the patient a great deal of distress the receptors in the vestibular apparatus may be destroyed by surgery or ultrasonic waves.

Headache

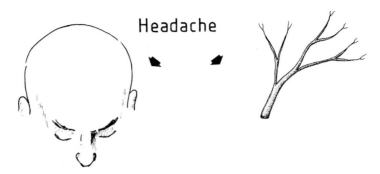

tension of scalp
muscles

change in blood vessel
calibre

Migraine

heredity   allergy

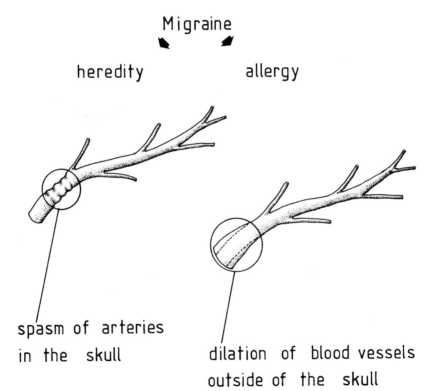

spasm of arteries
in the skull

dilation of blood vessels
outside of the skull

52　Headaches and migraine

Headaches do not arise from the brain itself or the overlying skull but occur due to tension in the scalp muscles or changes in the calibre of the blood vessels. Less commonly, they occur as a result of increased intracranial pressure, arising from a space-occupying lesion, or lowered intracranial pressure following a lumbar puncture. Hypertension and intracranial aneurysms cause vascular disturbances resulting in headaches, whereas worry and emotional disturbance cause muscle tension. After an epileptic attack there is frequently a headache.

Migraine

The cause of migraine is unknown although there does appear to be a hereditary factor. Other members of the family frequently suffer from allergic disorders, such as asthma or eczema. It is more common in women than men. The aura occurs due to spasm of the arteries within the skull such as those supplying the optic nerves. The headache is a result of dilatation of blood vessels outside the skull. Anything which alters the normal balance of the body, such as mental or physical stress, electrolyte disturbance, and hypoglycaemia may precipitate an attack. Menstruation, some oral contraceptives, and certain foods such as chocolate or cheese may bring on an attack. Some patients have a change in mood immediately before an attack but many may have a more tangible warning. Frequently this aura involves some disturbance of vision, there may be flashing lights, double vision or loss of part of the vision, and occasionally there is altered sensation on one side. This aura may be very short or last up to an hour, and is followed by a gradually increasing throbbing pain, the pain often becoming so intense that the individual is completely incapacitated by it. It is frequently accompanied by vomiting. The migraine may be over in a matter of hours or last several days.

If possible, precipitating factors should be avoided and at the first warning of an impeding attack ergotamine tartrate 1–2 mg, dissolved under the tongue, should be taken. The drug will act within an hour and if it does not it should not be repeated more than once as it may cause much damage. The signs of overdosage are similar to those of the migraine itself and therefore difficult to recognise. Rest in a quiet darkened room with aspirin based analgesics, a tranquillizer such as Integrin or Librium and if vomiting persists, Maxalon syrup or Dramamine suppositories. Clonidine helps to prevent attacks in some patients. Methysergide is also used as a preventitive agent but has serious side effects. Injection of sensitive trigger areas appears to help some people.